The Secular Prayers of Medicine

The Secular Prayers of Medicine

Stories from the Frontlines

Kateland Kelly, PA-C

HYPATIA
PRESS

Published by Hypatia Press in the United Kingdom in 2025

ISBN: 978-1-83919-647-8

www.hypatiapress.org

This book is dedicated to my herd of zebras, spoonies, and broken-hearted warriors: You are not alone and I'm glad you're still here.

Contents

Introduction by Father Nathan Monk

This book you now hold is neither a Bible nor a prayer book. There is nothing sacred about the words written here, by me or the author. Yet, as I read these words, it was clear to me that this collection of stories is the perseveration of a tradition based in antiquity that might still have a space in modernity. Kateland has neither demystified any faith nor created a new one with this work. Instead, she leads us on a journey toward the salvation of an ancient practice that has consistently gone in tandem with our attempts at science: to pray.

Prayer, in and of itself, is not a spiritual practice or an action exclusive to a religious institution. In the most ancient understandings of the word we now call prayer, we find its etymology rooted in not the heavens but in digging, thinking, making judgments, or engaging in conversation. These are not exclusively religious practices but the work done in every hospital around the world. Doctors and nurses dig for understanding, they make the best judgments they can, and through conversation both with clinicians and patients alike, they seek understanding.

Even the stages of grief are a type of prayer ritual where we must go from denial to acceptance. The object is to work through this process of loss in an almost liturgical way until one is able to reconcile this new reality they face.

With this book you will find yourself on that journey of reconciling the negotiations we all make in time or crisis or doubt. Prayer is not simply a negotiation with some historic deity to raise the dead or heal the sick. It is also prayer as the weeping mother pleads with the doctor for any diagnosis other than that their child has cancer, or as a patient must now grapple with a new prognosis. We can bow at the altar of the life support machine as we finally hear the sound of a flatline and beg for some different truth than this. One could even argue that the patient self-advocating with a doctor who seems to be missing something is akin to the stories of old as the prophets pleaded on behalf of their people.

These are the modern stories you will find here in The Secular Prayers of Medicine. These are the tales of guttural pleas that emit from us when all reason has failed and we have found ourselves backed against the wall of uncertainty. So, as you adventure through this world that Kateland has invited us into, there will be moments of discomfort, familiarity, and times you might wish to scream amen, a word that quite simply means, "So be it."

As you read this book, I'm sure that you will find yourself, as I did, more often than not saying amen. That final stage we must all excel to when we reach the end of our abilities, when we face loss, or uncertainties: acceptance of reality in all its chaotic beauty.

From the desk of Father Nathan Monk

Prologue

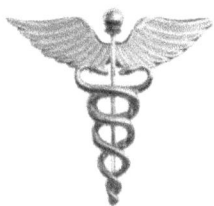

Impatient Patients

Patients are losing their patience while lobbing insults from the
lobby:
They are wondering what in the health is going on.

"What's taking so long?"
One woman wonders while the paramedics stroll past with the last
bed that can't breathe anymore,
But she's tapping her foot.

"Why aren't you better staffed?"
One man muses while I screw up my courage to shut down my frus-
trations and move onto the next medical mystery.

"Why does this cost so much?"
When you put a price on patients, you create costs that can't be cal-
culated at first
And while the rich get richer
All I can do is burn out and burn up
with this anger that just won't quit
because if I quit

that's it.

No more questions about time.
No more questions about staff.
No more questions about cost.

Because if I stop showing up, you'll start falling down
And you won't stop falling
Until you've landed squarely six feet under all the dirt you've been
throwing my way.

Secular Prayers

When we are most desperate in our times of medical need, we fall into secular prayers.

You might not call it praying.

Most of my patients don't recognize it when they're doing it.

I didn't realize that's what I had been doing all these years, myself.

That's because I'm not talking about the kind of prayers that are enshrined by pristine robes, stained glass windows, or offerings of water and wine. Those prayers are clean and structured. They are accompanied by a discrete wipe of a tear and a crossing of the heart. I have spent a lifetime collecting the secular prayers of medicine, and I have borne witness to those who actually answer those prayers.

I am writing from the perspective of an agnostic Physician Assistant who has danced with death multiple times and returned to tell the tale. When I first started practicing medicine, I thought I did so because I wanted to diagnose myself. I wanted to know why I was born in a body pixelated with pain and, despite decades of medical evaluations, no one could tell me why.

This collection of clinical cases kissed with personal poetry and storytelling opens a door into that world of prayer that can only be seen by the astute clinician who speaks the language of loss. Each of these chapters is based on a true story, though clinical cases have been fictionalized and patient details obscured to protect privacy (except when given explicit permission to share). These tailored tales are juxtaposed with my own journey to diagnostic deliverance and a dose of American medical history for context, all while exploring how storytelling impacts survival.

These cases include the type of praying where you fall to the ground, covered in shit, piss, blood, and tears, and cry it all out on a porcelain floor begging for salvation.

It's the kind of praying a mother does when her child is diagnosed with cancer and she finally punches the bathroom mirror.

It's the kind of praying a father does when he wipes the vomit from his chin and gets back to work because he needs to put food on the table.

It's when a girl gets her first period and watches a rose bloom in the bottom of a swirling drain while a blossom of shame germinates in her heart.

It's when a boy shuts the shower curtain closed around him, terrified his parents will scold him for touching his own body and punish him worse than the last time they caught him.

We might not know what to call it, but over the years in my medical practice I've been witness to all kinds of secular prayers. I'd like to invite you to read along and see what happens when our prayers are answered by a clinician who listens.

Why I Killed Myself

I never suspected that when I tried to end my world, the rest of it would try to join me.

Further, I never suspected I would turn into the type of ghost who guides others into this new plane of existence, and yet, here we are suspended in unprecedented times.

Growing up, I heard tales of how miraculous my survival to date truly was, all things considered. It only made sense that I confronted my mortality at a much younger age than my peers. I've struggled with my identity for as long as I can remember because it was defined for me before I could even cry.

I'm what happens when a "miracle child" not only survives, but grows up.

Born with a cardiac deformity, I experienced cardiac arrest, and death, twice before 12 months. My teen years and my 20s brought emotional anxiety along with an unruly immune system, requiring a near decade of oral chemotherapy and steroids to tame my wayward cells for a diagnosis of Autoimmune Hepatitis. I became an expert in living with an invisible illness, a master of masks, and an authority on emesis bags by the time I was sixteen years old.

I knew how to survive the world of chronic illness, but I didn't know how to actually live my life before the world ended. As I watched the world tumbling through a viral catastrophe sitting in near-total isolation in rural Vermont, I couldn't help but feel like I successfully killed myself the previous autumn and was sitting squarely in Purgatory.

Three months before the first recorded case of the coronavirus (COVID-19) in the United States, I placed my stethoscope in its original box. I was losing my physical footing with chronic illness, and it was taking its toll on my mental health. Despite surviving and compartmentalizing my childhood traumas, obtaining two advanced degrees, and successfully practicing medicine for a decade, it was in my 30s, when I was diagnosed with gastroparesis, that I truly, finally gave up.

Gastroparesis is simply the symptom of a paralyzed or slowed gastrointestinal system and includes a spectrum of gastrointestinal disorders with unclear etiologies. In my case, my stomach was paralyzed resulting in my inability to eat normal food for over three years, but no one could tell me why. No one could tell me if this unusual medical presentation had anything to do with the unusual medical presentations I experienced as a child and, as I was left to my own devices, I grew increasingly desperate.

As my mind, body, and hope wasted away, I found myself without the appropriate medical or mental care, and I considered suicide. As it turns out, I just didn't have the stomach for it.

I didn't want my life anymore. I didn't want to stay wrapped up in so much pain, and my world became nothing more than clocking in and checking out, taking care of patients while I let my own body crumble. All the while, I was experiencing systemic abuses both as a provider and a patient until one day, it was just too much. I resigned from that seemingly respectable clinical position because I was resigned to figuring out whether or not I wanted to live in this world anymore.

I gave up my white collar and became a ghost.

As I worked through my personal demons in therapy, I started to see my afterlife as less of a purgatory, less of a hell, and eventually something that felt comfortable.

I was gliding through my afterlife with ease, but then the world exploded and the COVID19 pandemic of 2020 put the entire world on pause. Everything changed into something contagious and sterile all at once.

The world turned into something everyone around me struggled to understand, but to me, it was so very familiar. The idea of constantly being afraid you might catch your death if the wrong person coughed in your direction is something that anyone with a suppressed immune system can understand, but the general public lived in blissful ignorance in the before times.

Individuals who live with chronic medical conditions that aren't easily perceived are a hardy bunch: We call ourselves the Invisibly Ill. Within the medical community, however, we're called Zebras. Zebras refer to a rare or unusual diagnosis, and I like to remind my colleagues that hypotheticals happen and we deserve dignity, even though most providers will assure you that "Zebras don't really happen that often." Just because you aren't looking and diagnosing us, doesn't mean we aren't there.

While my community of disabled individuals battened down the hatches with grim determination, we watched the healthy complain and obstruct the road to community safety. So often the healthy do not understand what sacrifice means until it happens to them. So often the living do not know what they can survive. But I do, and I've been documenting my story, and all the others that have crossed my path, because there is strength in knowing others survived. After several years of navigating the pandemic, the secular prayers are finally ready to be released back into the world.

I'm hopeful I can hold a lantern for the rest of the lost souls looking for their path on the road to recovery. This road to health and wellness is paved with good intentions and failed interventions, but by sharing our stories, I strive to show you examples of hope.

Sometimes our secular prayers are answered.

Student Years

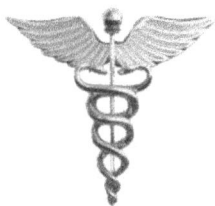

Rotting Out His Head

Monsters are not born; monsters are made, and doctors have a long history of creating monsters with diagnoses they can't contain.

A diagnosis is a powerful concept, capable of changing the entire course of a person's life, but, when a patient is *mis*diagnosed, their story can transform into a living nightmare. The History of Present Illness, or HPI, is arguably the most important part of a medical evaluation, and it's one of the first approaches a medical student needs to learn because this is the essence of your patient's story.

Simply put, it's a description of the patient's present illness starting with the very first symptom up until what brought the patient to you that very day. As you can imagine, HPIs can be very difficult to take mostly because every patient has a different communication style. Knowing what questions to ask is why we spend so much time training; we are honed to recognize patterns using keywords about the patient's state to guide our physical exam, assessment, and plan.

As a second-year physician assistant (PA) student, you were expected to see patients first to collect their history and obtain a basic physical exam. You'd then present your findings to your attending physician or instructor. Often, your instructor would then ask about your tentative plan and, if they approved, you would continue to the next medical case while that one was "cooking." If they didn't approve, you were in for a lesson. Some instructors were kinder than others.

Listen, report your findings, and learn.

Students who are not receptive to criticism or those who are hesitant to let the patient lead the conversation will struggle with obtaining accurate histories. So much of the question is how you ask it.

This was the reason I was drawn to medicine: the art of capturing the story.

As a teenager, I became increasingly ill and, to my frustrations, none of the medical providers seemed to listen to my story. My symptoms were dismissed and documented in a series of yes/no checkboxes that could never contain the complexity of my life, and so I was misdiagnosed over and over again, resulting in delayed care. It took me thirty-five years to get the correct diagnosis and ultimately the clinician who diagnosed me, was me.

When the medical history is ignored or edited to fit into an insurance-based narrative, patients suffer. As a twenty-two-year-old medical student, I was still ill, and in fact I was still on my oral chemotherapy at the time, but I was ready to learn how to capture my patient's story with respect and dignity from my elders.

Enter: Doctor Jackson.

He was a former PA turned MD and a phenomenal teacher, so when I landed in his rural hospital, I felt immediate kinship. He exemplified what I found so fascinating about emergency medicine: do not harm but take no shit. His drawl was southern comfort which, by the bedside, could make or break an experience, and you didn't want him to turn sour on you. He was a calm instructor and emphasized proper presentation when training his medical students.

On our first day together, he asked me what I liked about emergency medicine. I told him I enjoyed gynecology and psychiatry.

He asked what I didn't like so much and, in my foolishness, I answered honestly, "Anything to do with the eyes. I get a little queasy."

"You'll be seeing every eye complaint that walks in those doors." He announced it to the team.

No discussion.

No arguments.

My fate was sealed for the next four weeks: I would be the eye guy (gal).

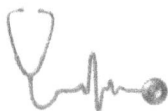

We worked in the step-down unit of the Emergency Room, which meant we were seeing the Urgent rather than Emergent patients. These often included individuals with lacerations, fractures, and an assortment of infections that wouldn't wait for their primary care provider. I found quickly though that the concept of having a PCP was one fraught with medical ableism and classism. In rural Virginia, we were often the PCP, specialist, and coroner all in one.

A patient's room turned green on the electronic board that broadcasted our patient load and that was my cue to go get a basic HPI and physical. It was go time.

40 y/o M: Red Eye – Right

I sighed, put my stethoscope around my neck, and steeled myself to enter the room.

The diagnoses flitted through my mind as I prepared a differential.

Conjunctivitis, iritis, blepharitis, foreign body...

I chanted the words, medical mantras, hoping that I would land on one of the easier itises. Those usually required an antibiotic prescription, a little patient education to wash the hands a bit better, and off they went into the night. I prayed that was all I'd have to deal with this time, so I could move onto the other people's puzzles I found more fascinating.

He sat, facing the door, and immediately my eye was drawn to his left eye, not the right. Sure, his right eye was red, but it was his left eye that was disgusting. I couldn't actually see his eyeball but I could hear it making squishing sounds from across the room. What I could appreciate was a glistening mass of flesh that looked like a meatball in the center of a plate of spaghetti. Except, this meatball was left out at room temperature for two weeks, and the spaghetti was turning into liquid under those lashes.

My mouth opened and I squeaked out, "I'm Kateland, I'm a second-year physician assistant student and I'm here to get your history. Can you tell me what brought you in today?"

The words came out quickly because I was spitting out the script I had memorized, but I was NOT listening to the patient. I wasn't even in the same room as the patient, truth be told, I was taking a deep dive into the dinner plate that used to be his left cornea.

Here's the thing though: Taking a history is all about focusing on the patient's words and while this is something I pride myself on now, this patient is a great example of how I got distracted by the physical exam first.

"Yea, my eye's all red and shit last couple of days." He blinked the ruby red 'good eye.'

"What about the left one?" I offered tentatively.

"This one don't hurt."

Normally this is where the clinician steps in with a series of seven questions that define a well-documented history of present illness:

Location: Where is the site of the problem?

Quality: What is the nature of the pain?

Severity: On a scale of one to ten, ten being pass out, how bad is the pain?

Duration: How long has this been bothering you?

Timing: What were you doing when it first started bothering you?

Modifying Factors: Does anything make it better or worse?

Associated signs and symptoms: Anything else bothering you?

Providers can go into so many different questions depending on those patient answers, but this is a good place to start. The reality is that, with this particular patient, the seven elements of the HPI went out the window as I struggled to formulate an approach.

What the actual hell is happening to your eye and why aren't you more scared??

That last question was more of my internal instincts kicking in and less of what I was taught during my didactic year, but it was definitely being posed in my mind. Why wasn't this man more upset? Because truly, he looked more bored than anything.

Before I could verbalize any of the pertinent questions I was supposed to be asking, he took his dominant hand and wiped at his left eye. The spaghetti eye.

A chunk of slimy skin fell into his lap.

I blinked. He did not.

My eyes stared at the piece of flesh that was now sitting on his torn jeans. The left eye oozed a little serous, straw-colored fluid with just a kiss of red.

"Did that uh, hurt?" I stammered.

"Did what hurt?"

"That." I pointed to the piece of necrotized flesh.

He wiped it onto the floor. "No, I already told you that one don't fucking hurt. Are you going to do anything 'bout the one that's fucking left or what!?"

"Uh, ya. Yea, lemme get my doctor."

As I left the room, I realized that man was in a lot of danger. I couldn't communicate my differential or the ultimate diagnosis though because I was too overwhelmed by what was the most disgusting eye I've ever seen. It was absolutely infected, that much I knew, but how or why I failed to capture.

I ran over to my attending and blurted, "His eyeballs' rotting out of his head."

Dr. Jackson smiled, not unkindly, but reprimanded me, "You can do a better HPI than that. Present him properly."

"Yea, uh, right ok. Um, 40-year-old African-American male, presenting with a red right eye of two days duration but his left eye is a mess. It's…It's rotting out of his head."

He chuckled but that did not calm my concern.

"No really, Doc, you need to get in there. I don't know what's going on, but his left eye is really messed up. I think he needs IV antibiotics, maybe surgery?"

"What's the diagnosis?" Dr Jackson asked calmly.

"It's an abscess!" I yelped.

Doctor Jackson led me back to the room. His bedside manner was significantly more measured than mine and I still channel his approach during times of stress. He said surprisingly little, nodded a lot, and quickly exited the room. The story was simple and unfortunately very sour. He was a homeless individual who was known on the fighting circuit, but one night a fight went wrong. His opponent ruptured his left eye and while he did have surgery, he did not have the means to follow up with outpatient care.

The surgical site became infected.

It then abscessed.

An abscess in the face is a real big deal. You don't need to be a medical provider to know that having a giant collection of pus less than an inch from your brain is a scary proposition. My gut instincts were correct; this man needed surgery.

But, he was stable.

I had all the time I needed to get the story before running up the rung.

Ultimately, this gentleman boxer of the streets was airlifted to a larger city hospital to receive the surgical and medical care he needed. Like so many of my patients, I never found out his ending, but he taught me the importance of taking my own vital signs before assigning a plan to a patient.

Providers panic, of course we do, but with practice we can keep those internal monologues screaming silently while we offer bedside interventions with compassion and composure.

Dr. Porno

"It's not a UTI," I informed the frustrated woman atop the stretcher.

"Then what the fuck is it?" she snapped at me while clapping at her two pre-teen children to stop making noise.

"I'd like to suggest a pelvic exam. Could we perhaps talk privately?" I motioned to her children with my eyes. I can't diagnose what I can't examine.

When a patient enters a medical office with a sensitive complaint, sometimes we need to provide distractions for family members to get them out of the room so we can conduct a physical exam. Mothers carrying for children don't always show up for their medical care, but, when they do, it's often a too little, too late sort of situation. In this case, a twenty-five-year-old mother of two was concerned about a urinary tract infection after reporting painful urination over the weekend.

She refused any testing beyond a pregnancy and urine screen.

Thankfully, the first was negative, but to her confusion, so was the urine screen.

"That's impossible! It burns down there."

I nodded again and motioned to one of my nurses to take the two kiddos out of the room for a little food adventure. Nurses always know where the best snacks are kept, and I don't care who you are or how old you are, if someone offers you chocolate and the chance to escape an emergency room bay, you will follow them wherever.

"You've got about five minutes before my nurse brings them back, so tell me what you've got to tell me now."

She didn't need to be told again. The true story came out in a waterfall of expletives. She was a BBW (Big Beautiful Woman) and she considered herself a bit of a Craigslist Kinkster. For those of you not familiar with the former online hookup hotspot, Craigslist once offered a digital space to put personals. Sometimes these personals were so sexual in nature, they were breaking the law, which is why the site eventually put the kibosh on those kinds of posts. Anyway, she would put up a post with a body shot, and she did have a very ample body pushing approximately four hundred and fifty pounds, and her address.

Whoever showed up to the party, showed up.

This was clearly not the safest sexual setup and, while it's not part of my job to judge, I was seriously concerned. Before I could ask her if any of her partners shared any recent infections, she blurted out:

"Well, I've been fucking a whole bunch of dudes and I don't know them, but I had a few over last week and I fell asleep after they were done fucking me."

So, no.

She did not know any of the men, so she consented to testing for a panel of sexually transmitted infections. We were going full swab! She agreed to the pelvic exam with a hefty sigh, warning me she didn't tolerate them easily because of her size. She told me she needed a metal speculum because if I attempted to use a disposable plastic one, it would simply break in half upon the first dilation.

When conducting pelvic exams, you need to take into account a woman's past emotional and sexual history, as well as the intricacies of the actual physical manipulation. Speculums hurt. If you've never experienced an inexperienced clinician giving your clitoris and labia a once over on the way to the subtle cervix, you don't know pain. As a woman, I was acutely aware of how embarrassing and uncomfortable a pelvic exam could be, so I wanted to approach her, and all my patients, with compassion.

As a student, my attending physician needed to be present for anything invasive, so after I finished presenting my concerns to Dr. Jackson, we grabbed two nurses and headed back to the room. The lithotomy position describes a woman lying on her back with her legs bent and spread open. This is the position we use for adult women for pelvic exams, but this patient posed an accessibility problem: She had a large pannus.

A pannus is a fold or flap of skin that overhangs the abdomen when morbidly obese. These areas can act as breeding grounds for infections because they harbor sweat and dead skin cells which then feed bacteria and even fungi. If it's dark and wet enough for long enough on the human body, you will germinate a yeast infection; that's just basic science.

As I settled between her spread legs, Dr. Jackson positioned himself behind her stretcher and the two nurses flanked me so they could each grab hold of her pannus. I needed two assistants to hold her abdominal fat up and out of the way so I could find her vulva.

When I did, the most impressive green froth bubbled out from her pink, hairy lips. I was not wearing a mask (and that represented the last time I did that!) and, when I looked up at Dr. Jackson with a slight panic in my eyes, I was grateful her mound obstructed her view of what the nurses and I were doing. As I struggled to swab the green waterfall spilling out onto the pad beneath her, the nurses and Dr. Jackson started gagging silently.

One of my superpowers, as I like to think of myself as your friendly neighborhood physician assistant, is that I have a significantly reduced sense of smell. This is secondary to a medication side effect from when I was treated with immunosuppressants during adolescence, but it sure has come in handy at the bedside. This was one of those times.

As we scooped up the swabs, we quickly excused ourselves and Dr. Jackson complimented me on my ability to keep a stone-cold face while he and the nurses, admittedly exaggeratedly, struggled with the smells. He asked me what I thought the pathology would show and I quickly spouted off a differential that included far too many possibilities. The green could be secondary to gonorrhea and the frothiness could be trichomonas. As for the white chunks in the folds of skin leading to the vulva, that was clearly a candida infection, I told Dr. Jackson. My treatment plan for her included a round of antibiotics, an antifungal, and a discussion on sexual safety.

I don't kink shame, but I will kink-educate.

Not only was I on the money about the gonorrhea, yeast, and trichomonas, but this poor woman also had chlamydia. It was time to break the news that her urinary burning was not a kidney infection, but a series of sexually transmitted infections. Luckily, all could be treated with the medications I mentioned earlier.

I went back into the room, holding her results in hand, and once again had one of the nurses distract the children with delectables.

I should have known something was amiss when she started typing on her cell phone, instead of responding to me. Instead of making eye contact with me, she furiously tapped away while muttering about the "fucker" under her breath.

"Ma'am?" I asked tentatively, taking a step closer to her. "Ma'am, would you like me to—"

Before I could ask for her consent to treat, she threw the phone up toward my face so that, in all its pixelated glory, an ebony member seemed to leap off the display and smack me upside the cheek. I had never, ever in my life seen an erection quite so erect. I'd never seen a penis so…plump. I coughed and choked as she yelled:

"This is the bastard; this is the fucker that did it to me! He tore a hole in me with his dick!"

Pure suspended silence enveloped the room as I had no words, but that didn't stop her from continuing, "I'm going to go right back to jail after I'm done killing this motherfucking devil dick."

I am ashamed to admit I split. I ran from that room, face bright red as a tomato as my Oma (grandmother) used to say, and tears running down my cheeks. I locked the employee bathroom but not without a flurry of fuss, as it was right across the nurses' station. The clinical staff was worried about me. I looked as though I was crying hysterically, so Dr. Jackson tapped on the door nervously.

"Kateland, you OK? What happened? Are you OK?" He questioned.

"I...I..." Gasping to catch my breath, I opened the door a crack, and giggled, "I need...to compose...myself."

I couldn't stop repeating the words *devil dick* in my head and it became this repetitive inner monologue that just left me laughing at the pure silliness of the alliteration. I just needed a few minutes and, thankfully, the ER staff completely understood this case of giggles.

He laughed and nodded as I finally spit out the basics of the story, and he closed the door knowingly giving me a full fifteen minutes to get myself together. This marked the second patient that had me out of sorts with Dr. Jackson, but this time, it was excused because it was objectively hysterical. Outside, the nurses had already figured out what happened, and they too were giggling. As I exited the bathroom, face freshly splashed with cold water, I was greeted with cascades of laughter and a brand-new nickname that haunted me for the remainder of that rotation: Dr. Porno.

I reminded them I was a physician assistant, but from that point on, they christened me an honorary doctor of dick, a healer for hookups, and a sage of sexual escapades!

After that case, I got all the sexually transmitted infections (which were often fun because we deconstructed stigmas) to the sexual assaults (which were difficult as a survivor myself). As for this case, the patient was treated appropriately and she had a great sense of humor about the entire visit. I apologized, while administering a high-dose antibiotic in her backside, and she told me to not take anything too seriously. She reassured me she wasn't actually going to kill him, and she'd consider screening sexual partners before playdates in the future. Her suggestion not to take anything too seriously is a good reminder. True to her advice, she spent the rest of her visit shaming that man by showing anyone and everyone the offending male's member.

After she was discharged, the final consensus of the ER staff was that his member was, in fact, the largest motherfucker they had ever seen.

Lights, Camera, Action

If you've never had a man look you dead in the eyes and proclaim that he wants to kill you, I can assure you it's quite a terrifying experience.

As I advanced through my student rotations, I found myself enthralled with the world of emergency medicine and with it the high emotions that accompany these cases. I opted for extra months in emergency medicine and gynecology, but found myself really shining with my mentally ill patients, even the ones that wanted me dead.

We just jived.

Psychiatry is one of those fields where you either love it or hate it and I've found, over the years, that many clinicians lack the empathy and patience required for caring for the mentally unstable. I know pain and I know what it feels like when people look at you like you're crazy. It sucks.

As a young girl, I was filled with anxiety.

First it began as typical nightmares, but they kept getting darker and more vivid. By the time I was six or seven, the nightmares shifted into night terrors and were accompanied by sleepwalking. I was nocturnally disassociating from the age of seven onward and my parents, in their unintentional ignorance, thought I was merely experiencing normal childhood dreams. They did their due diligence, though, and repeatedly brought me to my pediatrician. My symptoms were continually dismissed.

They told my parents that this was a normal part of childhood.

That nothing was wrong.

Everything felt wrong and no one listened.

I didn't have the words to adequately describe what I was experiencing at night. I found myself losing the ability to verbalize anything at all when I had a bad dream because I'd wake up in such states of overwhelming fear.

I'd jolt awake screaming, nightmares dotted with visions of demons, aliens, and monsters, but when my eyes were jolted open, they were still there in my physical bedroom. Sometimes they would fade within a few seconds of waking, but sometimes it was like a jump scare from a horror movie. If I closed my eyes tightly and focused on my breathing, eventually the night terrors would fade but I'd still be left a sweaty, shaking mess.

Then came sleepwalking. The episodes started harmlessly enough, but progressed to dangerous activities where I would wander the house and physically act out against those around me.

One time, I walked into my parents' bedroom and hit my father, screaming, "Where are my fucking cigarettes?"

No one in our family smokes, but my mother smartly advised me they were under my pillow, and I returned whence I came. Advising sleepwalkers that what they are looking for is "under their pillow" is a remarkably effective strategy that the pediatrician did impart upon us. However, a different time, I walked into my parents' bedroom and hit my father's side of the bed, again, and promptly announced as a thirteen-year-old girl, "Guess what! I'm fucking pregnant!"

I was not.

I had a lot of nightmares about being pregnant. They got worse as the years went on.

This is normal, reassured the pediatrician.

Nothing is wrong, reassured the pediatrician.

I was getting worse.

No one listened.

My parents took me to a neurologist when I was in middle school for a brain scan called an electroencephalogram when I started experiencing convulsions that mimicked epilepsy.

It was never epilepsy. If I knew then what I know now, I'd understand that mental illness never happens in a vacuum and that humans are miraculous creatures. We can sublimate emotions into the most unexpected of ways. For children, that can come out at nighttime in the form of parasomnias. That's what I experienced.

Parasomnias, the medical term for episodic behaviors that intrude into sleep, are most common in preschool aged children and frequently decrease over the first decade of life. Mine did not.

My mother made the grave error of asking the neurologist if thirteen-year-old me could get some Valium or Xanax because that had helped during a particularly violent episode that landed me in the local emergency room.

We were no doubt written off as drug seekers.

I learned to stop talking about the images that played out in my head each night when I closed my eyes. I also learned that there are some things you can't talk to anyone about, not even doctors.

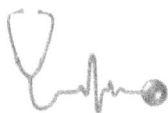

"What is the first thing you will do when we let you out of your restraints?" My voice trembled.

I was working my inpatient Psychiatry rotation when the Emergency Room paged for a consultation for a frequent flier. A well-known-to-the-psych-team paranoid schizophrenic was in the ER lobby informing the receptionist that it was a very "special night," but that he needed to be admitted as quickly as possible before he killed anyone to "celebrate."

Dr. Raj was my attending for psychiatry, and he was a very kind physician. He spoke with a light tilting accent that I found incredibly soothing, as did his patients, and he had a habit of smiling even when people were confiding in him about the worst things imaginable. It was the kind of smile that made you more comfortable talking.

I was one of five medical students rotating on his team at the time. The other four members shared cultural heritage with Dr. Raj and would often slip in and out their shared languages, whereas I was stuck languishing in the English word. The first week I rotated with them, they decided to treat me to a traditional Indian lunch to welcome me. I should have known something was amiss when they kept joking with each other while conveniently avoiding our common tongue. Each of them held their breath as I dug into my first bite of curry and then erupted into volcanic laughter when my throat turned into magma. The mango lassi drinks did not, in my humble opinion, help at all.

After that initial hazing, I was part of the team and it was a great group, although I packed my own lunches from that point onward.

So when this case came through in the early morning hours before dawn, Dr. Raj smiled and told me to take the lead as the other residents had already met our blood-thirsty individual during previous episodes.

Being a consulting specialist in a hospital is nice. You get paged when interesting cases come through the ER and, if they are admitted, you round on them. During that very same rotation, we had a variety of schizophrenics that were already in the inpatient unit, so I knew our ER bed would be in good company. My favorite pair of schizophrenics were Jesus and Satan, two gentlemen that had religious delusions that landed them on opposing moral sides. They were not related; they just happened to be in the unit at the same time, and they shared a conjoining wall.

When we'd round on the Jesus schizophrenic, he would offer to bless us. He'd hold his hands up, close his eyes, and mumble a prayer over you. He was nice. All the students wanted to meet Jesus. Most of the students regretted meeting Satan. Whereas Jesus would welcome you to his room with a smile and rarely needed any kind of restraints, Satan was usually tied down to the bed and prone to spitting. He'd curse you when you entered his room unless you pledged your soul to him, and I've got to give him this: he had great aim.

He would hock a loogie and then scream in delight when they landed, insisting he was, "Baptizing you in the name of the Almighty Evil."

There were other individuals on that unit that stuck with me, including a Black woman who had killed three people but couldn't remember the details. She was hospitalized at the time for urosepsis but, because of her delusions, she was still restrained to her bed with not one but two police officers posted outside her doors. I felt sad for her because the first time we spoke, she cried and explained that she never wanted to hurt anyone, but the voices wouldn't let her rest. She didn't fight against the restraints; she just melted into them with a sense of resignation I couldn't understand until decades later.

No matter how you slice it, consults from Emergency are pretty packaged up by the time the specialists arrive, and you generally know the diagnosis and disposition. When I entered into this schizophrenic ER bay, I found myself face to face with a thirty-year-old white man with a very grizzled brown beard and very sharp teeth strapped to the gurney.

Restraints, both physical and chemical in nature, are powerful.

If you've never been tied down to a hospital bed before, I sincerely do not recommend it. Any sense of dignity goes out the window. But patients should be restrained if they represent a danger to themselves or others. He was very clearly a danger.

"What's the first thing you would like to do if I were to take you out of those restraints?" I asked.

If a patient admits to wanting to hurt staff, they are going to get a one-way ticket to the inpatient unit. You have to establish how deep they are into their delusion without encouraging it, which can be a fine line. He smiled but didn't speak.

I repeated my question, "What is the first thing you will do when we let you out of your restraints?"

He stared at me intently and licked his lips. His teeth glinted brightly under the fluorescent lighting and he smiled sweetly, "I would rip your throat out of your body and drink your blood. I would kill you and I would eat you."

My stomach dropped. My heart flipped. I felt a little clammy.

I was safe though. He was struggling. I could help. I could listen.

He cocked his head to the side and whispered, "I'm a were-wolf."

I thought vampires drink blood, not werewolves, I mused wondering about the specifics of his fantasy. As we chatted more conversationally, he shrugged against the straps the best he could and said he was a very hungry wolf.

"OK, sir, in that case, you're getting admitted tonight." I smiled softly, my own teeth likely glinting in the lights.

"I know," he said. He started doing a little vertical happy dance against the gurney. "Thank you. I don't want to kill anyone tonight, but it's a special night and I have to celebrate."

And he *did* know he needed to be admitted. True to his history, he stopped taking his medication and, in the months leading up to his latest episode, he was eagerly awaiting a movie premiere but became increasingly obsessed with the plot. The night he presented to our unit he decided he needed to pick a moviegoer and drain them of their blood. He knew this was not socially acceptable, so he came to the hospital asking for help. As we wheeled him to the inpatient unit upstairs, he kept telling staff how excited he was to see all his friends back on the floor.

He couldn't wait to tell them about his adventures.

He couldn't wait for someone to listen.

Viagra Two Ways

When Viagra hit the United States market in 1998, it was an instant success even though erectile dysfunction, or ED, was not recognized as a medical condition at the time. It's been quite interesting watching conditions rise and fall over the years, but the jettison of erectile dysfunction as an accepted and widely marketed condition was what started mass medical marketing to the general populace.

Over 40,000 prescriptions were written within a few weeks of receiving FDA approval and it quickly became the fastest pharmaceutical to hit 1 billion in sales. Originally developed and patented by Pfizer in 1996, the little blue pill of sildenafil was meant to take care of pulmonary hypertension. This is a very specific kind of elevated blood pressure within the vessels of the lungs, and it can be life threatening, but the men in the study were interested in it not for their hearts, but for their hard-ons.

This is one of the cases where medication side effects overshadow the original clinical indication, and then marketing overshadows everything.

I've always been interested in marketing.

You could say I've been working in marketing my entire life, having started at the tender age of two years old. Before I delved into the world of diagnostics and after my cardiac arrests during infancy, I was an adorable toddler. I was so adorable, in fact, we were able to successfully monetize my appearance and my ability to verbalize by hooking up with an entertainment agency. Katie's Kids managed my commercial career and, over the span of about two years, I booked numerous local and national campaigns in both print and video media.

My favorite, and most successful, booking was Life cereal in 1988.

It was ten years before Viagra would hit the market, and Mikey, the original character developed by Life cereal, was all grown up. He did not die after ingesting Pop Rocks and soda, despite the modern myth that persists with him. The company behind the cereal wanted to capitalize on the nostalgia of Mikey and encourage the next generation of kids to give his favorite cereal a go, so they created a commercial series of children repeating the phrase, "Even Mikey liked it."

I got the lead role because my tiny tongue could vocalize, "Mikey was always an advocate of excellence."

I was paid in cinnamon cereal.

And money, there was money, but to be honest, as a child I was more into the idea of eating handfuls of cereal when I was on the shoot. Working as a commercial and print actress was a formative experience for me. I learned about movie magic, how to move products, and how to move my face in a way that would emulate the emotions I was supposed to be showcasing. I learned how to cry on command. I learned how to find the light. I understood how to copy words from a script and then translate it so that, when I looked at the camera, the audience melted. When the audience melts, they fork over their money.

Taking the train into New York City for shoots was always a highlight for me. We'd drive to the train station, park our family minivan for the day, and, before hopping onto the speeding silver bullet, I'd be allowed to choose one candy from the ticket shop.

It was always a Kit-Kat for Katie.

It was time to stop modeling and acting when the casting calls started calling for body modifications. Once, I was up for a toy commercial, but because the princess had brown hair, they were asking my mother to dye mine for the job. She asked me if I wanted my hair to look like the princess. I shook my head and said I liked my hair the way it was. She told me I wouldn't get to play with the toy for the shoot if I didn't. I shrugged and said OK, and that was that. My mother never pushed me into the commercial world, and it wasn't for lack of opportunistic requests. My mother considered acting to be a hobby and, while it was great that I made money and memories, if it wasn't fun, there just wasn't a point in pursuing that hobby.

Years later, as my interests transitioned into finding a way to stay alive (and make enough money to keep me alive), I felt a resurgence of interest in my childhood career. I applied for an internship at a pharmaceutical company, and then I maintained a relationship with them well through graduate school by working remotely in market research. Originally hired under an internship, I was quickly assigned to two pipeline products. During this time, many changes were happening in the world of medical marketing, including a huge backlash for some companies as they were accused of buying doctors and creating medical conditions for profit.

Our company was working on a female sexual stimulant, and we were actively trying to create a diagnosis called Female Hyposexual Desire Disorder for our drug, so the consumers weren't entirely wrong, in my humble opinion.

While I loved working on anything that had to do with sexual education and empowerment, my feminist inclinations had me questioning the marketing approach. Wouldn't it make more sense to address the underlying causes why women weren't feeling sexy?

Maybe they weren't horny because they weren't being listened to in the bedroom?

Maybe they weren't horny because they had a bad partner?

Regardless, pharmaceuticals are going to push forward if those who make them think there's money to be made, so we kept trying. We even developed diagnostic criteria to share with medical providers; we called it educational information on how to address low desire for women. When one of the team prepared for a conference in Florida to "educate the public about" about Hypoactive Sexual Desire Disorder, she expected a warm welcome.

I anticipated a slightly different response and I was right: Feminists didn't want our drugs.

They accused our company of medicalizing normal human behaviors.

They weren't wrong.

Which brings me back to Viagra because this drug transformed the way medical care is distributed in the United States. What makes this drug a unique case study in the world of American medicine is that it is often single-handedly acknowledged as transforming the world of direct-to-consumer pharmaceutical advertising. It debuted one year after the FDA relaxed the requirements for pharmaceutical companies to advertise directly to patients, and the timing was epic.

Those commercials with the smiling men and teeny-tiny prints at the bottom warning you of explosive diarrhea and death? Well, those are just part and parcel of American healthcare now. But prior to 1998, patients needed to talk to their medical providers for medicine. Patients didn't come into the clinic asking for brand name Band-Aids. Instead, they went into the clinic with symptoms and asked for the clinicians' expert medical opinions. What makes the case of Viagra even more interesting is that, while most drug trials last approximately ten years for safety and efficacy, Viagra completed those requirements in under two years, and continued to have trademarked success until 2003 when the FDA approved two competitors, Levitra and Cialis, flooding the market with options for impotent men.

We went from a cultural comfort level of not talking about sex to discussing erections during prime-time television because Pfizer knew that, to change medical marketing, they needed to create a need in the market. They linked impotence, which at the time wasn't recognized as a medical condition but rather a symptom, to the conditions doctors cared about: heart disease and diabetes. If you tell a clinician that the presence of erectile dysfunction can foreshadow a cardiac event eighteen months in advance of the danger, they're going to listen. Pfizer successfully medicalized a symptom for profit, and they created a blueprint for hundreds of drugs to do the same exact thing decades down the road.

Pfizer officials knew they had a tricky task with making impotence easy to talk about, so once they developed the medicalization of impotence as a diagnosis on the clinicians' side, they decided to go after the consumers directly next. They concluded they would not only talk about sex and impotence, but they would also hire the manliest man they could imagine to talk to their customers for them.

Enter celebrity medical spokespersons.

What man could command the attention of other men who wanted help in the bedroom but didn't want to admit to a flagging stamina?

Bob Dole.

As a former spokesperson for cereal, I can understand why they went for him. You want the customer to be able to place themselves in the position of the spokesperson and you want them to feel comfortable, portrayed, and confident in their medical decisions. In order to get into the stonewalled minds of heterosexual men, Pfizer officials decided that Bob Dole, senator, former presidential candidate, and respected war veteran, was the perfect person because he was so incredibly vanilla.

In his 1998 commercial debut, Dole looks at the camera wearing a power suit and red tie while stately instrumental music plays and calmly says, "It's a little embarrassing to talk about ED, but it's so important to millions of men and their partners that I decided to talk about it publicly."

Powerful.

Let's break that one sentence down from a medical marketer's point of view because, while it is a single, short sentence punctuated with music and dress, the whole set up is full of subliminal messages.

He acknowledged that asking for help with a sensitive subject is embarrassing. Because it is. He continued the discussion by identifying its importance to millions of men. It's not just about a lonely guy anymore, it's about connection and community and you don't feel so weird if you know there is strength in numbers. This technique is how we set the groundwork as marketers to normalize talking about lifestyle medicine. Lifestyle medication is any elective medication to treat a condition that could otherwise be managed by lifestyle adjustments. Bob Dole even brings the partners into the discussion so that now the conversation is about reconnecting with your spouse. That legitimizes the drug as a medical treatment and not a party favor meant for sexual deviants. Finally, the power suit and the instrumental music add several more layers of respectability and authority that men are trained to respond to since childhood.

Bob Dole and Viagra changed the way we talk about medicine.

So, imagine my surprise as a physician assistant student when one of the doctors on my Family Medicine rotation had a conniption fit over a Viagra prescription request. I wasn't assigned to him, so I watched from the nurse's station. My mouth was open in shock but my tongue was paralyzed. I remember wanting to speak up but being unable to find the words. I wanted to defend the patient. I wanted to tell the doctor he was a bigot but I didn't have any authority as a rotating student.

When I say he had a fit, I'm not just talking about how he refused to write the script; I'm talking about how he had a full-on tantrum. He was straight up offended when his male patient requested to try the medication during his annual preventative health exam.

I've also refused to prescribe Viagra, and I'll get to that in a moment, because over the years I've thought about this doctor often.

It was the slamming of the exam room door that got our attention. His medical assistant trembled, and in hindsight, I know now it's because she anticipated his reaction. The patient was an otherwise healthy fifty-something year old in a committed relationship, though at the time he wasn't married to his partner because it was still illegal in the United States. He was gay.

"Who scheduled that patient with me?!" The doctor's baritone voice reverberated through our bodies, "Who did it?"

He didn't wait for anyone to answer before he continued yelling so that everyone in the office from the back to the lobby could hear him shame the patient, "I am not writing a prescription for Viagra for some faggot."

Did he just call his patient a -

"Who thought it would be funny to do that? I'm not going back there. I'm not touching him again!" The doctor ranted, going so far as to hit a box of gloves toppling it off the station. "I touched him!"

The exam door opened, and a patient peeked his head out, obviously humiliated. That didn't stop the doctor from continuing.

"What kind of sick joke is this?" He went into his office, slamming that door as well, but not before we all watched as the patient heard him say, "He's disgusting. He can't get erections because it's unnatural. I'm not going back in there. Get him OUT OF MY OFFICE NOW!"

The patient listened in horror and, before anyone could close the gap between the nurse's station and his exam room, he quickly slinked out of the office using a back door. He literally couldn't face the lobby. I couldn't face the physician. I looked at my attending, but he didn't say anything. He kept his head down.

Everyone kept working.

That doctor refused to write a lifestyle medication for a man simply because he didn't approve of who he was. Never mind Bob Dole and his insistence that millions of men AND their partners care about this, you were straight out of luck if you weren't straight.

The reality is, as a primary care provider, you are responsible for the coordination of care for your patients from cradle to grave. That includes giving unbiased, respectful advice when it comes to sexual concerns. Pfizer literally changed the game for us as clinicians and yet this PCP decided to opt out of anything he didn't approve of morally. That's unacceptable in medicine. The fact he was angry that a gay patient was scheduled with him was discrimination then and it remains discrimination now decades later. Full stop.

Years later, I refused a Viagra script in my primary care practice and, to be fair, I did have a little bit of a fit over it.

It was a Friday night, and I was chilling on the couch with my partner when my cell phone started to ring. I didn't recognize the number, but it was a local one, so I picked it up and answered. This was before the days of unending collection calls for my medical debts, so I was still in the habit of answering random numbers.

A slurred voice sparkled through the line, "Heyyyy! How you doing?"

"Who is this?" I looked down at the phone perplexed, as it was after ten in the evening and I didn't recognize his voice.

In the background, I could hear laughter and clinking of glasses. It sounded like whoever was calling me was having a pretty good time, and wanted the party to continue. The cacophony of nightlife continued over the phone, so I repeated, "Who is this?"

He stated his name and, with surprise, I realized he was a patient from our office!

"So anyways, can you call me in some Viagra for tonight?" His request was surprisingly slur free.

I blinked. "No! What? No!"

"Aw, come on! I just need one or two for tonight. I'm not far from the 24-hour pharmacy." He continued, completely unaware of how inappropriate it was to be calling my cell phone after hours for a medication request that I've never prescribed to him before.

Also, I wasn't on call.

Also, and most importantly, how the hell did he get my cell phone number?

I asked him as much and he informed me that my personal cell phone number, along with a few of the other clinicians' details, were posted in the employee break room and, because of this, he figured he could call any of us anytime. It was clearly an oversight, but he didn't know that.

Our clinic had a call service that would screen patient calls overnight. They would only be patched through to the provider on shift to triage via a text message if they met certain criteria. By giving the provider the details via text, we could get to a private location and call the patients back after blocking our numbers. This is how we maintained our privacy while also maintaining continuity of care. It's also how we kept our providers sane, so we weren't constantly barraged by requests better suited to daylight hours.

Denying this Viagra request was not based on moral judgment, though I *was* judging him.

I was judging his lack of boundaries, but I kept my reaction to a minimum on the phone and waited until I hung up to start my hysterical tirade. I hooted and hollered until my partner and I laughed with tears in our eyes. He jokingly accused me of cockblocking my patient and gatekeeping sex but agreed that was appointment-worthy. My patient was drunk, happy, and hopeful, but I ultimately dashed his spirits by telling him to schedule an appointment with me during business hours.

I may have cockblocked him, but I coordinated his care.

When he did finally come in for his annual preventive exam, we found out he was both hypertensive and a Type II diabetic requiring medication management.

I guess Pfizer was onto something after all.

Circumcision Syncope

I've never been a fan of routine infant circumcision.

Then again, I'm also not a fan of piercing infants' ears.

I just can't get behind chopping off the tip of a functional organ when it's done to a nonconsenting child.

The United States is the only developed country to circumcise male infants regularly for nonreligious reasons and it represents a fairly lucrative elective medical industry. Circumcision rates vary according to religious affiliation, insurance coverage, hospital type, and socioeconomic status. If you have health insurance, you may only pay a copay of sixty dollars, but if you are a self-pay family, the average price for a newborn circumcision can go up to $800. This gets a little funky when age gets into it because Kaiser Permanente, for example, will only cover costs for circumcisions performed on newborns, but will not cover it for older children and adults unless it's medically indicated in the cases of infections or cancer.

At the time of this writing, circumcision rates are highest in the Midwestern states, with 74% of the male population boasting snipped skin, whereas they are lowest in Western states, at only 30% of the population snipped. The general rates of circumcision are highest in non-Hispanic White Americans at 91% compared to 76% of non-Hispanic Black Americans and 44% of Mexican Americans.

In 1996, the Canadian Pediatric Society (CPS) issued a clinical practical guideline that stated, "The overall evidence of the benefits and harms of circumcision is so evenly balanced that it does not support recommending circumcision as a routine procedure for newborns."

Two years after I graduated Physician Assistant school, in 2012, the American Academy of Pediatrics (AAP) task force on circumcision of the male infant concluded: "The health benefits of newborn male circumcision outweigh the risks; furthermore, the benefits of newborn male circumcision justify access to this procedure for families who choose it."

The AAP cited specific benefits including prevention of urinary tract infections, HIV, or other sexually transmitted infection acquisition, and decreased risk of penile cancer, and the American College of Obstetricians and Gynecologists (ACOG) endorsed these conclusions. The AAP went on to further state that male circumcision does not seem to adversely affect penile sexual function, sensitivity, or satisfaction, though I can't help but wonder *HOW* they reached those subjective conclusions.

In that same year, 2012, the American Urological Association (AUA) reaffirmed their 2007 statement that outlined, "…neonatal circumcision has potential medical benefits and advantages as well as disadvantages and risks…It is generally a safe procedure when performed by an experienced operator…when circumcision is being discussed with parents and informed consent is obtained, medical benefits and risks, and ethnic, cultural, religious, and individual preferences should be considered. The risks and disadvantages of circumcision are encountered early whereas the advantages and benefits are prospective."

My Pediatrics rotation was done under the tutelage of a Dr. Bishop and his Physician Assistant, both of whom were devout members of the Church of Latter-Day Saints (AKA Mormons). They practiced within the bounds of their beliefs, which I quickly found was common in Utah but I appreciated they both kept an open mind when teaching an agnostic such as myself.

They put me at ease right away, asking me what my comfort level with the LDS Church's beliefs were. They let me lead the conversation. Interestingly enough, I was able to respond with a positive story that had all of us smiling with the seemingly divine coincidences.

On my flight out to Utah, I read "The Idiot's Guide to Mormonism," gifted to me by my then-boyfriend. He grew up in the LDS Church and, although he left, his family was still very much active. This initially provided somewhat of a divide, as I had no intention of converting to such a religion, but over time his family accepted that he, and I, are good people without their god. Either way, it is important to be respectful, and so I took out my book and placed it in the front seat pocket before the flight took off.

As I watched the seats filling, I prayed mine would remain empty.

Even before the pandemic the idea of being in a plane was bothersome to me because of being so close to other people. Listening to their breath, and, worse, listening to them chew, was mind-bogglingly painful for me. I always, always prayed for empty seats. As the steady flow of people turned to a trickle, I thought I got lucky until an elderly white man in that stereotypical white shirt, black tie, black pants motif started ambling to my aisle. He sat down next to me and smiled politely. At first, I hesitated to reach for my reading material but eventually boredom got the better of me.

He was unwrapping a brie and turkey sandwich when the back cover caught his eye.

"We don't believe that, you know." He wiggled his white caterpillar eyebrows at the book.

"Which part?" I flipped to the back cover, trying to guess which byline he was referencing.

"Polygamy. We don't do that."

"Oh, I know. The FLDS still practice it though," I responded.

He nodded sagely, "Want half of my sandwich?"

I did. I really did. Brie and turkey sandwiches are a favorite of mine and the airport food was so expensive that I had opted against anything other than the complimentary pretzels and room temperature water. Student life! Before I could answer, he handed me half of his sandwich and proceeded to give me an impromptu lesson about the history of the church. He shared that he was visiting for their General Conference, and not just as a practitioner of belief, but as one of the religious authorities. I was in for a truly unprecedented philosophical discussion.

When he found out I was on my way to conduct my Primary Care, Pediatrics, and Obstetrics and Gynecology rotations, he shared he recently lost a sibling to pneumonia. He went from answering my questions about his religion to asking me if there was anything that could have been done differently for his sister.

To reflect that he asked me earthly questions about medicine and mankind was sobering and a compliment. I reassured him that he did everything he could and he asked if I would pray with him. I did. It was the first time I experienced a secular prayer with a stranger, though I didn't realize it at the time. Even though he was an authority figure to millions of Mormons, he was just a frail, old man who missed his sister. He was still wondering what more he could have done and still asking for medical providers to absolve him of his survivor's guilt.

I answered his prayer and absolved him of his survivor's guilt even though his religion answered none of my prayers.

I spent a lot of time out West learning about the LDS Church. Most of my patients there were devout and, overall, were quite kind to me. I will say that, for most of my time out in Utah, it felt as if, when I got to know a Mormon, there was a hopeful undercurrent that they could convert me, since I was not a member of their club.

Once one woman grasped my hand tightly as she confided, "The light of Jesus is in your eyes."

It wasn't.

My relationship with religion is complicated. I am not a Christian despite attending Catholic school from elementary to college. I am a convert of nature. I recognize the divinity that is Mother Nature, and will spend my time worshiping at the altar of lakes and ponds, not the ones with wine and white bread.

Either way, the two Mormon preceptors taught me how to use a patient's religion to your advantage as a clinician. Dr. Bishop would engage patients with the Word of Wisdom, which refers to dietary recommendations set forth, unofficially, by the Church of Latter-Day Saints.

I can't tell you how many times I called out the devout diabetics for overeating Krispy Kreme by asking them, "Would that fall under the Word of Wisdom?"

One day, both of my preceptors were smiling a conspiratorial grin, and I knew something special was on the schedule. A few days before, they had treated me to a medication reconciliation of an eight-year-old girl who was on Viagra; I got major credit for properly identifying she was a pulmonary hypertension patient without getting tripped up on the erectile dysfunction indication. It's rather common for attendings to throw you into cases expecting you to miss something, and then they use it as a successful teaching moment.

"What?" I asked as they welcomed me into their shared office.

"Ready to assist with your first circumcision today?" Dr. Bishop asked, and I groaned.

He knew I was in the camp of avoiding medical interventions unless necessary, and avoiding cutting your children's genitals at birth. Both men shared they were circumcised, and they didn't remember it and said, "It really isn't that bad."

I side-eyed them and resigned myself to the morning's fate. I'd learn how to circumcise.

Before the infant arrived, they went over the procedure with me, and I spent some time watching videos in anticipation. It's not a complicated procedure, but it does require a steady hand and a lot of confidence. The standard approach for an outpatient circumcision, and what we did in that office, was a combination of oral sucrose and a dorsal penile nerve block. The dorsal penile block is done with lidocaine but not epinephrine, as use of epinephrine is associated with loss of penile tissue. Further, it is best to administer the nerve block with a single injection to minimize the risk of penile swelling.

Once a baby is undressed, they are placed into a papoose, also known as a Circumstraint. I couldn't describe a Circumstraint any better than they can, so enjoy this blurb of copy they put out to market their medical device to offices:

"...in less than thirty seconds, a nurse can immobilize the struggling infant securely in the correct position with the Circumstraint. The immobilizer works on a proven principle of positive 4-point restraint. Soft wide Velcro brand fastener straps encircle the infant's elbows and knees, depriving him of leverage. The child is held safely and securely without danger of escape. Circumstraints comfortably contoured shape positions the infant, hips elevated, perfectly presenting the genitalia."

Any time bondage is involved in a medical procedure, my eyebrows shoot up.

I felt lightheaded before we even left our office to go to the procedure room.

Seeing the Circumstraint had my blood pressure up as I waited for the nurse to bring momma back with her baby boy. The mother, a young Hispanic woman with round cheeks, came around the corner with the nurse and she promptly thrust her son into my arms.

I'm often quite awkward with babies and this was no exception, "What are you doing?" I asked instinctively.

"Take him, I'll be in the lobby," she replied. Mom started to turn on her heels without so much as a pause.

"Wait, aren't you going to be in the room to soothe him?" I wondered.

"Nope! This is my sixth son. No way I'm in the room to watch that." She shook her head and galloped off to the safe lobby. I looked down at the mewling infant in my arms, face already pink with frustration, and I walked him into the surgical suite.

I felt like I was bringing a lamb to slaughter…*Can you hear them, Clarice?*

Both men were in good spirits, laughing with each other and smiling happily at the baby boy. I stood to the left of my doctor and observed. As they pinched his penis, I felt myself get a little clammy. As they injected the lidocaine, I got a little weak in the knees. As the first bead of blood bubbled up, before the clamp was secured to the prepuce, my hand reached behind me, reflexively searching for a chair.

"You going down, Kelly?" Dr. Bishop asked with a laugh.

"Yup. Like a ship." I backed away until I found the wall. I slid over to a chair and I told myself I'd never do a snip as I faded to black.

The Biggest Little Dragon

After I woke up from my thirty-second snooze with the circumcision, Dr. Bishop spent the rest of the rotation laughing at my lack of stomach for the situation. I decided against scrubbing in for anymore snips, but I committed to discussing the procedure with my patients' families with unbiased information.

Moving beyond circumcisions, I used to wonder where penis issues and related insecurities originated in grown men, because they certainly weren't born with them as children. This next patient case still remains a core clinical memory because it's where I realized the importance of proper terminology for body parts in a very physical way.

When lessons are doled out with pain, you pay attention.

Sometimes, penis issues are directly instilled into kids by their parents.

Some parents are uneasy with anatomy and just generally uncomfortable with the idea of the human body. This is especially true when they think of their children in the context of puberty. Some parents simply cannot stand saying "penis" or "vagina" (especially vagina). Some parents decide that it makes more sense to circumvent these words entirely by replacing them with cute nicknames or outright gibberish, but as a clinician, this only makes my job harder, because it strips me of a neutral language for educating as the child ages.

This type of wordplay ranges from the basic "wee-wee" and "pee-pee" to the more flamboyant and fantastic, as this one family illustrated so many years ago. Using immature language can seed a poor relationship with the body, and contribute to medical misunderstandings later in life. I've seen grown adults argue with me over why Saran Wrap is an acceptable alternative for condoms, even as I'm holding their positive pregnancy tests. I wish it were an exaggeration, but it's not.

A young mother, accompanied by *her* mother, brought her five-year-old son in for his kindergarten well check. This visit is both fun and fearsome. It is fun in the sense that you get to play with a five-year-old to assess their mental and physical development. This includes games with clinical relevance, such as asking the child to draw a person and playing Simon Says with active range of motion. It's a lot easier to do a scoliosis check on a kid if they think they're winning a game.

This visit also traditionally includes several vaccines, and I was going to administer them.

Vaccines shouldn't be controversial, but, for as long as I've been practicing medicine, there has been a growing movement to abdicate this branch of science. I am a skeptical person by nature when it comes to man-made interventions, and I prefer a natural approach to most concerns, but vaccines are one of those modern medical marvels that save lives. Unless you have a true medical contraindication, vaccines are a crucial part of a well child check.

Thankfully, this mother consented to the full panel of vaccines and reassured us they could help hold him down. I should have known this wasn't going to work out before we even attempted the shots based purely on his physical exam. See, the shots come at the end of the visit, so that the crying child doesn't associate the pain with the provider.

He did a great job with all the developmental challenges, and he let me look in his ears without much fuss. He was less enthused with the genital examination and immediately put up a fight. It is my personal practice to never force a child to undress, and I let the parent take the lead on that. It's important for children to feel comfortable setting boundaries, but it's also important to detect medical conditions in a timely manner.

"Alright, mama, now we need him undressed for a quick genital check."

He frowned and stared at me angrily.

"Go ahead and show her your biggest little dragon! Go ahead, show her the dragon," his mom cajoled.

"What did you just say?" I wondered out loud, not entirely on purpose.

"That's his wee-wee." She smiled proudly and tickled his belly. "That's what we call it, right? The biggest little dragon! Now go ahead and show her your big little dragon?"

"OK! Rawr!!!" He growled at me as he pulled down his pants. "Dragon!"

I bit my tongue and conducted the last part of his exam just in time for him to growl once more as the nurse brought in the tray of vaccines. He was a full dragon at this point, though, and there was no going back. He continued to scratch and growl menacingly.

"Alright, mama, are we doing this or do you want me to have another nurse assist?" I asked.

"We hold, we hold." She assured me.

When vaccinating children, it's best to ensure they are secure and won't move during the injection. There's nothing quite so unnerving as bending a needle in the thigh of a particularly strong child, and we explain this to parents before we attempt the procedure. In this case, both mom and grandmother felt comfortable holding him. It's best when caregivers can be in the room offering a hug, so we proceeded at their assurance they were ready for this.

Mom took one arm, grandma took the other arm, and the nurse helped hold his contralateral leg. I readied the first shot, a muscular injection, and I braced myself for his cries as we rapid-fired multiple vaccines. With the first shriek, his grandma let go. With the second shriek, his mother let go, and with a final primordial scream, he kicked me squarely in the solar plexus.

I went down like a bag of wet potatoes.

My nurse cried out to the errant mother, "Why'd you let go?"

And the mom cradled her son, yelling at me on the ground, "You hurt my baby! You hurt my king!"

"King?" I wondered weakly. I thought he was a dragon, now he's a king, too?

King Dragon ended up getting his full series of shots that day, though another nurse stepped in to help hold him after his unintentional assault on my abdomen. His mother was indignant, and his grandmother was offended. But, by the time they left, they verbalized understanding that we were not trying to hurt him. Dr. Bishop reminded her that she consented to her son's treatment before we even brought the needles in.

We were just doing our jobs.

We just wanted the parents to listen to us.

As a parent, it is your job to frame your child's medical visits, because the way they relate to their bodies begins with these trips. Children are sponges; they soak up the information you present to them, as well as the emotional vibes you put into the environment.

If you don't think your child can handle their annual vaccines, what are you going to tell them when I diagnose them with cancer?

Bechet Dump

"We do not dispute historical diagnoses on this unit," Dr. Top stated firmly to our team of four internal medicine students. "John Doe has multiple sclerosis."

I looked at the middle-aged Middle Eastern man on the gurney, his mouth peeling where sores blossomed, his eyes glassy yet pained. He couldn't speak, but when he tried, it came out as a guttural groan. While he made consistent eye contact with us as we spoke about him and around him, he couldn't participate in his own care. He would repeatedly slam his head back against the pillow in frustration.

He had no voice.

He had no name or identification.

He had no friends or family we could contact.

That's not entirely true; he had a family. They just didn't want him anymore. He was dumped at the entrance of our Emergency Room, unable to walk or speak for himself and after two days of trying to find someone to take him home, the hospital realized that he was a "dump and run." We now had to coordinate his care because no one was coming to take him home.

Dr. Top wasn't up for a discussion. He was already overwhelmed and understaffed, and the last thing he needed was a bunch of medical students mucking up an already mucky hospitalist admission. If the chart said Multiple Sclerosis (MS), that's what the patient had, and we weren't going to play Dr. House to find a rare diagnosis, according to him.

I couldn't help but wonder how accurate a historical diagnosis is when the patient can't participate and the family is absent. How can we confirm?

Well, theoretically we can confirm with the physical when the history fails us.

While Multiple Sclerosis is the most common immune-mediated inflammatory demyelinating disease of the central nervous system, it can be very difficult to diagnose and manage. The typical patient ideally presents as a young adult with one or more clinically distinct episodes of central nervous system dysfunction with at least a partial resolution. That's a lot of medical mumbojumbo, so what does it actually mean to the average patient on the street?

Not a whole lot.

The symptoms of Multiple Sclerosis can be vague, intermittent, and easily dismissed by the average person. Even more so if the person doesn't have access to bodily education or an understanding of how to access medical care when things start to go funky. For example, MS can present with: sensory loss on one side, unilateral vision loss, double vision, gait or balance disturbances, vertigo, bladder issues, and pain. Individually, or even combined, with intermittent relapsing patterns it can be easy to see how even the most astute clinician can misdiagnose or overlook this condition.

If you're lucky as a clinician, not as a patient, your case might come in complaining of electric-like shock sensations that run down the back or limbs upon flexion of the neck. This is known as Lhermitte's Sign and should put you down this diagnostic pathway. Classically, symptoms will develop over a few hours to days, and then slowly yet progressively remit over the following weeks to months. It's important to remember that remissions may be incomplete, and patients may not return to their baseline functioning after each flare.

If John Doe were coming to us in a Primary Care or outpatient setting, things might have been different. If he came in with concerns of vertigo, for example, he might have been treated to a workup that started with a history. We didn't know when our John Doe lost the ability to communicate, or if he ever had it, but he was nonverbal, unable to write, and either did not know, or could no longer communicate with, sign language.

The cornerstone for diagnosing MS is a magnetic resonance imaging (MRI) during the first attack of symptoms, but that's not always realistic. It wasn't realistic for John Doe and now, as our team of students stared at him, blinking blankly, we didn't know where to go.

You see, the problem with John Doe was that his chart was pretty empty, and we steadily filled it with assumptions.

We assumed he had no allergies, because no one could tell us otherwise.

We assumed he had MS, because that's what matched his clinical presentation the best, according to Dr. Top.

We assumed he wanted everything we did to him, including admitting him to an inpatient floor…including placing IVs in him and administering medications he couldn't understand…and including tying him down to the bed when he got combative.

No one treated him like a human.

Everyone treated him like a piece of furniture, talking about him as if he weren't even there. When I teach medical students now, I teach the patient at the same time. I engage all parties around the medical bed and show them why we do the things we do as medical providers.

My mother taught me the importance of never talking around a patient.

My mom was in her early twenties when she was first diagnosed with Malignant Melanoma. She spent her childhood tanning with baby oil and tin foil wrapped record album covers, rocking out to the sweet tunes of The Mamas & The Papas and Aretha Franklin. When she should have been celebrating early marriage and planning her family, she was instead sitting in a doctor's office being told she needed surgery. She and my father were trying to have me, at the time, and this was not the way she expected to have her first major surgery.

Prior to going under anesthesia, she was warned she may be facing a lower leg amputation but thankfully, the surgeon was able to preserve her limb. The morning after her surgery, the doctor entered her room with a gaggle of students. While he preserved her leg, she still lost the inguinal lymph nodes and about eight inches by eight inches of muscle.

She was asleep when they entered her room, rounding on the surgical patients. Without warning the lights were turned on and she found herself staring down a team of about ten strangers, while the surgeon had removed her sheet and left her naked from the waist down.

The doctor didn't acknowledge my mother. He didn't ask for her permission for an examination with an audience. He didn't even make eye contact with her as he detailed the surgery to his medical students. He went so far as to say one of the reasons she didn't lose her leg was because "she was so fat to begin with it stopped it from spreading."

She scrambled to cover her genitals while the doctor continued detailing her case, mouth open aghast at the circumstances. When she finally gained her voice, she spoke up and told him to get "the fuck out of my room until you learn how to talk to patients."

In the days following her surgery, she experienced a miscarriage. She shared with me, they didn't test for pregnancy before surgery back then, even if the patient was a young, twenty-something woman. Back in those days, they let women figure it out on their own, so when she started passing big clots after missing her period, she realized it wasn't just a period. Her surgeon didn't acknowledge the miscarriage at her follow-up appointment outpatient. What he did do, though, was assault her one last time.

She told me that even though her surgical site was horrifically scarred and painful, and even though she miscarried her firstborn, he considered it a success. Before he ended the visit, he slapped her scar, hard, with right hand the way you would slap a piece of meat, stating, "I did a damn good job."

My mother remembers the sound of him laughing at her as he walked out of the room.

My mother's surgery, and cancer management, highlights how horrific it is when patients are intentionally excluded from their medical care: Informed consent no longer exists.

Now, some twenty years later as a medical student myself, I watched my attending talk about John Doe in a similarly detached manner and I felt generational rage. I felt my calling coming up in the back of my throat: do no harm, but take no shit.

I felt like we were harming this man by doing a whole lot of shit to him.

But no one could stop us, and insurance paid out because we were putting him up. And as long as protocol is tight, then the attending must be right, right?

At this point in my medical student career, I was taking oral immunosuppressants for a presumed diagnosis of Autoimmune Hepatitis. I was struggling with nausea spikes, so I took our lead Internal Medicine resident aside and told her if I ever needed to step away, I was tending to my side effects. Looking back now, I'm so glad I disputed my historical diagnoses because they were never quite correct. In hindsight, I also wonder if anyone looked at me the way I looked at John Doe when he was at his most reduced state.

Did anyone ever wonder if someone did me wrong?

As our team of students prepared John Doe for admission into the hospital, we conducted a thorough physical exam. We found he had significant ulcerations along his eyes, mouth, and penis. The sores were seronegative for herpes virus, and we couldn't identify a cause otherwise. This set off the lead medical students' radar, which is how Bechet's Syndrome was even brought up. The attending accused the lead student of hunting for Zebras and reprimanded her stating our only real job was coordinating his transfer of care to a long-term facility.

Bechet's, also known as the Silk Road Syndrome, is a rare autoimmune disorder in which your body attacks your blood vessels. Like many autoimmune disorders, it is likely that genetic and environmental factors play a role, but at the time of this writing, there was little attention paid to these unusual Zebras outside of the halls of rheumatology. Anyone living with autoimmune manifestations, myself included, would often be swept under the rug of a placeholder diagnosis and blasted with steroids until their body calmed down, proper diagnosis be damned.

Bechet's Disease occurs in less than 1,000 patients in the United States annually and is more common in people with ancestry from along the Silk Road, such as Turkey, Iran, Japan, China, and East Asia. While women can develop Bechet's Disease, it is more common and more severe in men's presentations and will often present around the second or third decade of life. Initial symptoms can be easily dismissed and can include:

Recurrent raised, round lesions in the mouth that turn into painful ulcers and take up to three weeks to resolve; this is the most common sign of Bechet's Disease.

Acne-like sores throughout the body or red, raised, tender nodules on the lower legs.

Red, open sores on the scrotum or vulva; these often are painful and will scar.

Inflammation of the eyes causes redness, pain, and blurred vision bilaterally.

Relapsing joint swelling, stiffness, and pain that last between one to three weeks per flare.

Abdominal pain, diarrhea, and bleeding can be present if digestive vessels are affected.

Perhaps most damning, right there in the medical texts, was the section describing long-term effects of untreated Bechet's Disease on the brain. Aneurysms, narrowing of the vessels, and inflammation can result in headaches, fever, disorientation, poor balance, and stroke. In a patient who had flare after flare, year after year, without access to medical education, diagnosis or management, it was very possible he had stroked out multiple times.

His imaging confirmed our suspicions. His gray matter was grossly gone, and it looked like Swiss cheese instead of functional tissue. It was coded as multiple sclerosis lesions, but we wondered as a team if the ulcers plaguing his eyes, mouth, and genitals were related to ancestry from the Silk Road. He was admitted and taken off our service, so I never found out what happened to the man with the red eyes and the lost voice.

I thought back to all the times I told my doctors something felt off, but it was vague, and I was dismissed. I thought back to my swollen joints, my autoimmune cross that I wasn't sure I should be bearing, and I wondered what would have happened if someone listened to me when I told them that my brain felt foggy, my stomach shocked me, and my joints were slowly turning to stone.

As I finished my rotations as a physician assistant student and applied to jobs as a licensed practitioner, this case remained with me. John Doe reminded me that we are all but one diagnosis away from devastation, and he became the first ghost to haunt me over the next few decades.

John Doe was powerless to contest his historical diagnosis but I was not. I hoped and prayed that with time and experience I would be able to not only contest my childhood diagnoses, but confirm the true pathology of my chronic pain.

Early Practice

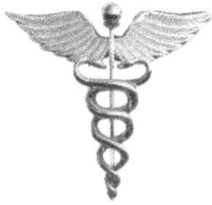

Early Practice

You Killed My Child

I always hated Christmas.

While other kids counted the days until Santa was dropping off dozens of presents, I was usually huddled around the toilet bowl praying I wouldn't lose another serving of sugar cookies. I wasn't praying to Jesus, the reason for the season as my Christian family and friends would say, but I was praying to someone else. Something else. My secular prayers went mostly unanswered. For whatever reason, Christmas was inexplicably linked to another mysterious "stomach flu" for me. Every year.

It was like clockwork.

I grew to hate the darkening of the days. Getting sick was just so predictable for the winter season it became a tradition of sorts. We'd stock ginger candies and gingersnaps, not because we were channeling cheer but because we were trying to minimize reflux. I'd expect to cancel celebrations at the last minute and really, I didn't mind it. At least, that's what I told myself over the years.

It wasn't until my fifteenth Christmas did the reasoning behind my vomiting change. It wasn't a stomach flu anymore. Then again, maybe it never was.

A few months before, the doctors told me to start taking little neon yellow-green pills for my acutely worsening joint and abdominal pain. I didn't know what my exact diagnosis was until that Christmas Eve, though.

When trying to describe my symptoms to my medical team, and my parents, I referred to the abdominal pain as "liver lightening" and the wrist pain as stigmata. It was a dull, deep ache in the bilateral wrists and hands that felt as though someone was driving nails into my body. The doctors didn't find my descriptions particularly helpful and more than one told me that I needed to describe my symptoms according to their pain scale and not some random religious metaphor.

But once I started taking the little neon yellow-green pills, my stigmata calmed down and the liver lightening became less frequent, but still ever-present. These were strange electric shocks that would originate from my solar plexus and stab into my liver. It felt like my organs were being fried up from the inside out. This pain would last for only a few seconds, but was accompanied by episodes of dizziness and decreased exercise tolerance.

The intolerance for exercise got so bad that I was excused from all physical education requirements in public school as far back as I can remember, including being allowed to walk the mile in grade school. My physical frailty had always been excused and dismissed as just a girl who's dainty. This new constellation of symptoms, however, gave me newfound freedom from physical work in school. I got an elevator pass and extra time between classes so I could creakily move without getting hit by other students in the hallway accidentally. Even tiny bumps to my body caused exquisite spikes in pain and bruises would bloom like black roses under my skin. Even now, my healing rate is quite delayed and I'm prone to develop keloids that keep track of my injuries.

There were so many tests leading up to the little yellow pills.

Blood draws led to ultrasounds which led to CT scans which led to liver biopsies which led to the little yellow pills but no clear diagnosis was shared with me. As far as I knew, I had medication to help the pain but it was treatment without a cause.

One morning when I was supposed to be getting ready for high school, I found myself unable to push the comforter off my aching body. I lay trapped under my blankets, panic rising in the back of my throat. Was this one of the night terrors? Was I still asleep?

I was awake, and when my father stormed into the room to find me, what he assumed was sleeping, he was none too pleased because we were all going to be late. Taking the comforter off of me, he grabbed my wrist and yanked. His eyes widened to match mine as my mouth opened in an "O" of pure pain; every single one of my vertebra cracked with the forced forward movement, and my wrist snapped under the pressure of his hand hold. He didn't apologize for yelling; he was too shocked. He didn't say anything at all as I fell backward crying in pain, struggling to understand why my body was turning to stone.

With movement, my joints slowly worked. It became a ritual to wake up early, nauseated before school, to sometimes vomit and always slowly stretch out my crackling body. Back in those days, there was no easy access to medical knowledge. No WebMD or Wikipedia for me to peruse. So, I learned the old-fashioned way:

Medical television and the public library

My favorite show was House M.D. which debuted two years after I started taking my little yellow pills. This American medical drama series ran for eight seasons and carried me through undergraduate and graduate school. The main character, Dr. Gregory House, is an unconventional medical genius who is warped with pain and addiction while still leading a team of diagnosticians at a fictional teaching hospital in New Jersey.

His bedside manner was atrocious and that was part of the draw of him as a fictional character. He was bitter because his disability was the direct result of a missed diagnosis and delayed medical care. I was just like House, I used to think, my diagnoses weren't right but I didn't know what the right answer was. Truthfully, I never idolized House for his misanthropic ways; I idolized him because I wanted to become like him. I wanted to be a gentler, kinder version of House, Lady House if you will. I wanted to be the one that diagnosed the medical cases that stumped everyone including mine. I wanted to answer the secular prayers that went ignored.

I wasn't the only one who fell in love with the show. Something about this show hit on an underlying current of dissatisfaction with American healthcare. While it could get corny at times, it highlighted the desperation of patients living with atypical case presentations and it led to increased awareness for many orphan conditions. House was among the top ten series in the United

States during its early seasons, and became the most watched television program in the world in 2008, the year I entered my Physician Assistant program in Virginia. Medical television combined with my descent into American healthcare as a patient in the 2000s led to my twin passions of writing and healing.

I found as long as I took the little pills that no one else was supposed to touch, the stigmata calmed. I still experienced liver lightning, but less often. The nausea never went away, and the vomiting got worse with the little pills.

My mother kept the pharmaceutical inserts close at hand, never allowing me to glimpse them, and I lacked any way to research them beyond what the doctor had already told me. The doctor informed my parents my symptoms most closely matched Juvenile Rheumatoid Arthritis though they wanted to rule out a few other rare diseases with additional tests.

Rheumatoid arthritis is a chronic, systemic, autoimmune, inflammatory disorder that primarily involves the synovial joints. The arthritis is classically symmetrical and most typically presents as a polyarticular (more than one joint is affected) disease with a gradual onset. Symptoms usually progress from the periphery and will result in significant disability and deformity within ten to twenty years of diagnosis, if not properly managed. These symptoms can affect patients' capacity to perform the activities of daily living and certainly affected my ability to walk, use the stairs, get dressed by myself, or even wash myself without help.

I can understand why they diagnosed me with this condition. Just like my Bechet's Syndrome patient, the symptoms fit well enough, so it worked as a placeholder. Morning stiffness is one of the more common features and is defined as, "a slowness or difficulty moving the joints when getting out of bed or after staying in one position for too long, which involves both sides of the body and gets better with movement."

My stigmata had a name! I took the pills like a good girl and secretly prayed that was all I needed to do to get better. It was on Christmas Eve when I washed my hair that my world exploded.

I took pride in my hair, my nearly knee-length golden tresses. I joked my hair was what would happen if Rapunzel and Lady Godiva had a daughter. Rapunzel was trapped in a tower, and I felt trapped by my body. As for Lady Godiva, she was a French nobleman who protested the mistreatment of the underclass by riding her horse naked through town to spite her husband. I always wanted to be that kind of badass woman who used her body to her advantage, not someone who cowered within its cages. Needless to say, when I could finally wash my hair without feeling screaming pain in my wrists, I was delighted and distracted from the fact I didn't know what I was taking or precisely why.

But on Christmas Eve when I washed my hair, the hair didn't stay on my head.

I screamed as my hair started falling out and I watched as it swirled around the bottom of the drain. I fell to my knees and punched the floor repeatedly, my hand collapsing under the trauma. Trembling, I wrapped myself in a towel, threw on my Christmas pajamas, and ran downstairs to find my mother sitting across from the lighted tree, tears in her eyes.

"What's happening to me?" I held out my hands with inches of golden strands hanging limply.

"The doctor said this might not happen." She pulled me in for a hug, "I'm so, so sorry."

"What might happen?" I gasped.

"Your hair. It's temporary."

"What am I taking? Mom! What am I on?" I rocked back and forth, unable to focus on a single thought but constantly barraged with images of dying. People dying of cancer lost their hair. "Do I have cancer?"

No, I didn't have cancer, my mother explained, but the doctors theorized that my body was attacking my joints, and they placed me on steroids to calm the inflammation. The little yellow pills were oral immunosuppressants because some of the tests, specifically the liver tests, suggested the root of my arthritis was actually Autoimmune Hepatitis and not Rheumatoid Arthritis like I thought.

It was oral chemotherapy. I never realized chemotherapy could come in a pill. I thought you had to go to a hospital and get hooked up to an IV to get chemotherapy. I thought you had to wear special protective equipment to administer it…and then I realized why no one else was allowed to touch the pills, why my mother needed to wear gloves when she cut them, and why my younger sister wasn't supposed to use the same bathroom as me.

"Why didn't you tell me? How could you?" I sobbed.

"I didn't want to ruin Christmas," my mother weakly whispered.

My first job as a physician assistant felt like Christmas every day.

I made my oral chemotherapy my entire identity which is eventually how I came to take a job in oncology. Beyond my personal experiences, my background in oncology pharmaceuticals made me a shoo-in for an inpatient/outpatient mixed position at a cancer institute. My heart did not sing when I read the job summary, but those student loans were due and money was the motivator that led me to accept.

Ultimately, that position reminded me too much of being a patient. The transition from medical student to being a fully-fledged practicing physician assistant is daunting. Despite training for years, there's still a sense of "What if I mess up?" and this is especially true if you throw yourself into a subspeciality field right off the bat.

Bobby was a teenager, but they were in our unit because they met the weight criteria for an adult transplant. They had a round face, from the steroids we put them on, and a perpetual smile, from their own personal reserves. Their family traveled to our institution because they prayed for an answer and God sent them to us. At least, that's what her father told me when he held my hand with tears in his eyes, thanking me for taking their case. They were a devout Catholic family and my last name hinted I was a devout Catholic girl myself, though I really wasn't. They found comfort in our presumed shared spiritual heritage and I prayed with them on several occasions.

Bobby was diagnosed with acute lymphoblastic leukemia (ALL). In medical school when studying hematology, my professor joked that "ALL children get leukemia". That quip always bothered me because one of the long-term side effects of my adolescent treatment regimen was leukemia later in life. Looking back, oncology was never the right place for me, but…money. That's really what motivated me to take that first position. Student loans were coming soon, and I didn't want to risk defaulting.

I also craved the respectability that came with saying, "I'm an oncologist."

Somehow, that felt bigger, better, and stronger than sticking to the primary care frontlines that I fell in love with, but again…money.

I felt overwhelmed in that position from day one. While interviewing, I was promised a robust training period, but the reality was I was seeing patients independently on call in about half the time I expected. I put my head down, found two mentors on site, and tried to soak up all the knowledge I could.

The lead physician was a cheerful person in front of patients, but in front of clinical staff he could turn caustic at a moment's notice. Where I struggled the most was his falsely hopeful pitch when proposing experimental treatment plans. Having worked in pharmaceuticals, I understood the process of pipeline-to-market testing and, in cancer, you do agree to be a guinea pig. But all these people believed they were the pigs that would be spared from slaughter. All of these people believed they would be spared from the worst complications if they just ignored the reality of the drugs they were on long enough and prayed hard enough.

The providers that remain in oncology know that miracles can happen but we are only human. We cannot save everyone and we should never pretend that we can.

Likewise, we must do our best to remain impartial and avoid assigning emotions to cases and patients. Transference is the medical phenomena in which a clinician identifies or sympathizes with a patient to the point of transferring emotions between each other. It's safe to say that I struggled with this for the first portion of my practice. I felt what my patients were feeling and, when it came time to take off the white coat and go home, the stories kept tugging at the corners of my mind. They kept reminding me of my inability to help or heal, and the shortcomings of medicine in general. The longer I found myself in oncology, the worse those feelings became. Eventually, all my cancer patients blurred together with the exception of one or two cases.

Bobby is one of those cases and they will always represent oncology to me.

They will always represent what it means to acknowledge your boundaries.

Bobby struggled throughout their treatment regimen. They suffered through many complications with grace, but perhaps the most punishing was when they developed horrific sores throughout their mucous membranes, including an infected anal fissure. I've seen grown men fall to their knees over lesser complications, but not this kid, not this sixteen-year-old. Their strength really inspired me, and so their death really destroyed me.

They passed away, quietly, from fungal pneumonia in the early morning hours. The rest of the team wasn't coming in for another four hours or so, but I was on call.

I could hear their father's screams before I got off of the elevator.

The nurses warned me that the father refused to leave the bedside and was becoming progressively more combative. Bobby's mother fainted and was resting with family in another room. I didn't want to go into the room where Bobby's father lay guard over their cooling corpse.

I knew they all bought the pitch that a bone marrow transplant would save their child, but the reality wasn't what they expected. I knew they nodded happily when we informed them of every risk, and I knew they were too distracted by the possibility of a cure to ever really consider the complications and the possibility that it wouldn't work. Every time we'd discuss a complication or try to explain why Bobby was worsening, they would wave us off and reassure us that God would take care of it. God told the parents that we were going to save their child.

"Just have faith," the parents kept repeating, "We have faith in you."

As Catholics, they struggled with the concept of a fetal bone marrow transplant because that was forbidden, but it was also their only hope. I also clung to high hopes for their recovery so their final examination, the death examination, was heartbreaking for me. As I checked their inactive pupillary reflexes and absent peripheral pulses, I choked imagining myself on that gurney. I choked remembering my hair falling out, like Bobby's completely did, of my body swelling from the steroids, like Bobby's did, and of it eventually becoming cold and hard, like Bobby's body did under my gloved hands.

The father kept beating his fists against the wall and, occasionally, against their cold body. The nurses tried to keep him from hurting himself and us, but it was no use. Several got injured in the process, but I am embarrassed to admit that I don't really remember much beyond the feel of Bobby's body under my hands.

We were often told that, when grieving family members lash out physically, it's just part of the job. Be smart, be aware, and get out of the way. Deal with it as a professional. He didn't land any of his physical strikes aimed at me, but his words branded me for life:

"You killed my child. You promised you'd save them, but you lied and then you killed them."

You Look Like Me

Having someone in authority that looks like you, is powerful medicine.

It's important to understand the kinship that happens between a patient and a provider when they look similar to each other. Humans naturally gravitate toward the similar; there is safety in numbers, and we are a social species. Whether you call them your family or your tribe, it is likely you have a group of people that you gravitate toward that look like you do, act like you do, and think like you do.

But the first time a patient accused me of being racist, I didn't know what to do.

I never really considered how race affected me until I started practicing medicine and then I couldn't *not* acknowledge it. I had transitioned out of oncology and into primary care where I met with thousands of patients from different backgrounds but this case took place in the South before I moved out West. Before I could even introduce myself to my elderly black patient, the visit went sideways.

This matchstick of a woman started screaming, "Oh no, no. I ain't letting no white girl touch me. Out! Out of here!" She shooed me with her purse, lips stuck together in a frown, "I ain't nothing but a n*gger to you."

It was like all the air was sucked from the room.

"Oh! No! I'm not from around here! I'm a Yankee!" I yelped in surprise, trying to distance myself from the established racism of the south as if my Connecticut culture could excuse me.

It did though.

Her eyes narrowed and she goes, "Shit, I'm from New York."

"My mom's from New York originally." I was more than a little scared of her outburst, and I offered common ground as a peace offering.

She broke out into a grin that looked like a busted picket fence, "Girl, sorry about that. Ever since moving down South, I've been dealing with these racist assholes. It's nice to meet another Northerner."

She sat down, slapped her knee, and the two of us spent a solid five minutes commiserating the racism that was endemic in that region. I told her that I didn't even feel comfortable whispering the "N word" so when she lobbed it at me when I walked in, I didn't know what to do. She laughed and thanked me for not being a racist "asshole" (her words, not mine).

Growing up in a proud German household, my Oma would tell us stories about her time in the war. She was a pre-teenager when Adolf Hitler rose to power and her father was a police officer in their hometown. My great grandfather was a renegade and, even though he was cloaked in respectability, like me, he wasn't afraid to use his privilege to the benefit of others.

He was not a true believing Nazi and he had a daughter with a defect to protect.

All children were expected to participate in Hitler Youth, and that included regular marching drills. My Oma did not care much for these marching exercises. She found the entire prospect of Hitler Youth to be boring and exhausting. The way she used to tell the story, she would much rather go swimming in the creek with her girlfriends and didn't understand why they had to salute a "funny little man with a mustache."

To circumvent my Oma's stubbornness and to keep his family safe, my great grandfather arranged for her to be evaluated by the family physician and proclaimed unfit to participate in marches. Why? She was born with a congenital heart deformity, at that time not clearly defined in the medical record, but one that both I and my niece were also born with many decades later:

Ventricular Septal Defect.

This was risky because sick children were not beloved by Nazi Germany but the risk was calculated and it paid off.

My Oma was deemed sick enough to not participate in the physical drills, but well enough to be allowed to continue her genetic legacy. Unfortunately for her, that meant that, while she had free time when the other kids were marching, it was spent sequestered indoors as a "sick kid." She missed out on swimming in the creek as well as running outside ever again.

My family was part of the resistance in Germany and eventually they fled after helping others escape first. My Oma created a life here in the States and went on to be one of my great inspirations in life, but suffice it to say when I think of my German heritage, it is a complicated mixture of pride and pessimism. Even so, decades later, when I go to special events, I bring my black medicine bag gifted to me on the day of my graduation by Oma, and I keep it in my office.

My heritage may define my ancestral past, but I choose to believe in the power of personal autonomy for creating a better future. For me that means practicing medicine with awareness and compassion, so that no matter who finds themselves on the exam table in front of me, they are treated with dignity. But sometimes the patients that ended up on my exam table scared me.

Just like the first time a patient accused me of being racist, I had no idea what to do when confronted with an actual racist.

His girlfriend was the one who arranged his physical. At the time, my office accepted self-pay patients and had a sliding scale of services including physicals for a variety of programs ranging from Boy Scouts to pre-operative clearances for cardiac surgery. This gentleman needed a physical for entrance into a residential facility, but the girlfriend wasn't very forthright with the details of where the facility was. She was very insistent on when it was needed, though.

Immediately.

As someone who lives with chronic pain, I understand that addiction is an unfortunate reality for many, so I prepared for his visit thinking I was getting him help with sober housing. I was so very wrong. When he arrived at the office, it was apparent he had muscular dystrophy and used the assistance of two walking canes, braced on his wrists, to ambulate forward in a quad-like fashion.

He was accompanied by the insistent girlfriend, a brunette in cut-offs, and she gently guided him at the elbow. His skin was pale yet sunburnt in a way I'm familiar with, but it was the dark ink covering his epidermis that held us all captive.

Swastikas. So many swastikas.

His third eye was replaced by the jarring windmill of hate and his head was shaved smooth so that it could be crowned by yet another swastika facing the sun. His arms were decorated in a variety of insignia that I didn't entirely recognize but knew were calling cards for neo-Nazis.

I was able to spy him from the quarantined comfort of my closed-door office, so my reaction was enshrined in that solitude. Glancing at the black and gold medical bag gifted by my Oma, I said a silent prayer to my ancestors for guidance and for strength. How could I confront this mirror of a man without letting my disgust show through?

I had only moments before my receptionist would phone me to inform me he was here, and I needed to switch gears fast. I reminded myself that tattoos are just ink. That I did not know this man's story yet, and it could be one of redemption. To remain calm, professional, and pick up where the chief complaint starts. Besides, he was here for entry into a residential facility, so perhaps he was putting his life back together after a difficult start? This was my fevered thought process. I tried; I really did.

His name was highlighted on my electronic medical record and the chief complaint was filled in dutifully by my medical assistant: Prison Physical.

Oh, shit.

I had done my fair share of prison physicals before. They do require a delicate touch, and it is my personal practice to avoid asking prospective inmates why they are going in, so the topic doesn't come up unless they explicitly offer it up themselves. Generally, these exams must be conducted within fourteen days of entrance into the system.

First and foremost, individuals should be screened for infectious disease when entering a correctional facility. This is as easy as grabbing a urine sample, blood sample, and in the post-pandemic world of coronavirus, a nasal swab. As this patient was going from the general populace to prison, he was in desperate need of coordination of care for his chronic medical problems. He was on several antispasmodic medications, a serotonin selective reuptake inhibitor, and was requesting a note regarding his copious alcohol intake because if he were to stop acutely, he would be at risk for withdrawal. Alcohol withdrawal can kill you and it is managed inpatient or in prison using a tapering system of various medications including benzodiazepines.

I steeled my nerves outside his exam door and knocked.

To my surprise, as I opened the door he struggled to stand and politely said, "It's nice to meet you, Doctor. Thank you for agreeing to do this."

I shook my head, pleasantly surprised, and slipped right into my clarification of credentials just as I would with any other patient, "Oh, of course. But I'm not a doctor. I'm a physician assistant."

We settled into the history portion of the visit, and he shared his medication list with me, and that his entrance date was only six days away. I could see why his partner was antsy on the phone prior. He was so polite. He was cooperative and seemed intelligent. He answered all my questions without hesitation and, while his girlfriend seemed to fidget at every other word, he remained surprisingly still. Perhaps he really was seeking a better turn in life, and I found myself glad I took his case. Just like any other patient, he needed medical care and who was I to judge him based on the color (or rather inking) of his skin?

Now I will ask potential inmates if they know about how long they will be gone. This gives me some idea of what they're dealing with emotionally if not outright letting me in on the scoop. He rolled his crystalline blue eyes and muttered he would be gone for a long time.

"It's bullshit," the girlfriend spat. "It's just bullshit. It's all technicalities."

"I don't need to know the details," I said, clearly trying to move on to the physical exam. Tensions were rising and I really didn't need to know the details.

His pink lips stretched to expose his yellowed teeth and I felt nervous. His girlfriend launched into a monologue about how he was "set up." I tried my best to focus on the physical exam. I silently prayed his offense was drug related.

She continued, "…they weren't even that young anyway, some of them were teens…."

It wasn't drugs. I had no words, but I motioned to the exam table, holding out my hand to help him up when he stumbled with his crutches. I focused on my breathing because I had committed to caring for him. What was another five minutes in the room? He stayed silent but she kept talking, except I only registered clips and phrases. But when the girlfriend said, "…they wanted it…" I fully disassociated.

My stomach clenched as I pressed down on him, watching the faint trail of fuzzy hair depress as my hands palpated his appendix and then his bladder. I don't remember much, but I remember an internal monologue floating over me. The voice inside my head was quiet, small, and feminine, and she whispered:

Just get it over with. Just go through the motions. Look past him and it will be over soon. Just breathe through it and it will be over soon.

I shook my head, repressing my memories. I was in no place to wonder about the details of the children he hurt; speculation can happen after examination and after documentation. As we concluded the physical exam, I prepared to turn him over to my nurse for a blood draw.

He took my hand and I flinched, but holding it firmly he said, "Thank you again for being so nice to me."

"Again, it's my job to take care of patients." I nodded, trying to extricate my hand from his and I realized, a case too late, that while it is my job to take care of patients, I don't have to take care of all of them.

"I knew you were a nice German girl." He smiled sickly and my stomach flipped inside out. "You look like me."

Prescribing Dream Control

"Can you help with nightmares?"

I asked the patient for more details between bites of Pad Thai as I answered the clinic telephone, attempting to sneak some food between cases.

When patients inquired about nightmares I would encourage a referral to a therapist. As you may remember, I have lived with nightmares, and night terrors, for the better part of my life, so I tend to perk up when someone asks questions about parasomnias.

Sometimes, parents would ask about medication control on behalf of children, but this patient threw me for a loop when she disclosed the specifics of her request. She wasn't actually asking about nightmares for herself; she wanted me to stop her boyfriend from having erotic dreams about her.

She had been dating her beau for several months, but they were an LDS couple in their early twenties and they had not yet decided to tie the knot. In the LDS faith, sexual relations before marriage are frowned upon, so as you might imagine:

Mormons marry young.

Really young.

The young men will leave their home for a two-year religious mission at the age of eighteen and, when they return, they are full of vim and vigor but they can't spend any of it unless it's within the bonds of marriage. Enter the virginal bride.

She felt passion toward him, but lamented that they couldn't act on it until marriage. In the meantime, though, he admitted his passion toward her recently manifested itself in the form of wet dreams.

I choked on a peanut.

"Excuse me?"

The patient repeated her question, her voice crackling hopefully over the phone, "Well, can you help stop his nightmares?"

My mind whirled, first contemplating the question from a clinical perspective before realizing the ethical implications. She wanted me to medicate her boyfriend so that he would not experience nocturnal emissions. She wanted him to "be a gentleman and to stop thinking such impure thoughts." This wasn't about parasomnia, nightmares, or anything similar: it was about controlling someone when they were unconscious – and it set off major red flags.

"No, no, I cannot prescribe anything like that." I shook my head. "But maybe the two of you would like to come in together so we can get you a relationship counselor?"

She wasn't interested, and she insisted I could prescribe something, "But I was reading online, there's this medicine you can inject and it lowers a man's sex drive."

As we spoke on the phone, I did a quick Google search to figure out exactly what put that thought in her head. The internet can be a wild place filled with bad ideas and worse interventions.

I thought back to my pediatric training when I first moved out West. It was there that I was first introduced to the weird world of LDS sex. When an entire group of people suppresses sexual education and doubles down on a religion that emphasizes making babies, things get a little funky. Over the years, I had several LDS mothers request a "wedding night exam" for their daughter the day before they were wed.

It's exactly as it sounds.

They would request a pelvic examination, with a speculum, not for a pap smear prior to the wedding but rather to help "stretch them out" the day before the deed. It was to help women with any pain that their husbands might make them feel by getting them ready. Open wide!

Never mind having a candid conversation with your partner about going slow and using a lot of lube.

Never mind discussing what feels good. Nope, just stretch 'em out and send them down the aisle.

But, getting back to our couple with "nightmares," I quickly found the source of the desperate woman's inspiration: Lupron!

Lupron, or Leuprolide Acetate, is a gonadotropin-releasing agent used to treat uterine fibroids, endometriosis, prostate cancer, and premature puberty. It is also used in rare cases to suppress the sex drive of violent sexual offenders, specifically pedophiles.

Side effects of Lupron include injection site complications such as redness, pain, and infection, as well as night sweats, insomnia, dizziness, testicle pain, and their strangely desired outcome: decreased sex drive.

When I asked the woman on the phone if her boyfriend wanted to stop having those dreams, she couldn't answer. And when I told her she was describing chemical castration, she was shocked I would suggest such a thing.

"I don't want to castrate him!" she explained.

"Well, what do you think you're asking me to do with medication? Suppress his sex drive? I don't know what else you'd call it."

Rather than decreasing her boyfriend's sex drive medically, I encouraged them to talk. She hesitated at first, partially because LDS women are not encouraged to take an active role in sex. She couldn't imagine talking about it with him. She was ashamed and indoctrinated by a lifetime of conservative culture and she was projecting those concepts onto him.

Together, we started to dismantle those projections, one telephone visit at a time.

We discussed what is and isn't healthy for a sex drive, the importance of listening to your partners when setting physical boundaries, and masturbation from a medical perspective. I also explained why nocturnal emissions happen. She listened, and she didn't force her boyfriend into a chemically altered state. They eventually married and as far as I know, they lived happily ever after.

Had she posed that question to a true believing Mormon clinician, I'm not certain what their response would be. I hope they wouldn't say yes to such a request, but over the years I've treated former Mormons whose families did worse to them. I had patients tell me tales of when they were mere teenagers, their parents arranged to have them captured in the dead of night from their beds. These children were taken out to the desert to rid them of their sexual deviations whether that be an inclination toward "same-sex attraction" as the LDS say, or masturbation. Some of these children eventually grew up to become adults who struggled with authenticity within their marriage. I had multiple queer patients confide in me that they felt like their love life was arranged by family expectations and not true demonstrations of affection between consenting adults.

Additionally, the citizens of Utah were incredibly concerned about pornography consumption. I can't even describe how many times a spouse made an appointment for their partner to address their "sex addiction". How many sex addicts did I actually treat in Utah? None. How many spouses got angry at me when I told them that sexual attraction to others doesn't disappear because the state recognizes your tax break? So many. Just because you don't like what your partner likes to look at, that doesn't mean that they are evil sinners.

My god, when will Christians stop judging themselves and each other?

When will they stop shaming bodies and funding shock therapy, waterboarding, and psychological torture?

When will they stop seeking medical absolution for actions they take which are nothing more than sexual abuse?

Sexual abuse can occur at any age and can be more insidious that the average person realizes. Practicing medicine in Utah gave me an intimate glimpse into sexual abuse that stemmed from a highly organized religious institution and, over time, I became more vocal in speaking out against the LDS church meddling with medicine. When you teach children to fear their bodies because they might "betray them with lust," you are sowing the seeds of sexual dysfunction by abusing them. When you teach adolescents that they can't touch themselves without fear of losing their temple card (and access to divinity), you are sexually abusing them. When you force twelve-year-old boys into closed door rooms with forty-year-old men to discuss their masturbation habits, you are sexually abusing them. When you force adults into conversion therapy because you don't approve of who they love, you are sexually abusing them.

Spirituality can offer some comfort, but not when it leads you to enforce your will on another's body. If you ask yourself for a prescription to prevent passion in your relationship, you might need to consider that you are perpetuating a cycle of abuse, and not love.

D.I.D. I Do That?

Generally speaking, I don't accept food from patients.

I've always been pretty picky about food. When I was a child, my Oma would make special meals just for me if I didn't want what the rest of the family was enjoying. She'd grill me lamb chops while everyone else ate meatloaf. She'd cook filet mignon and slice it for my lunches. I didn't enjoy peanut butter and jelly sandwiches as a kid, but I loved pairing brie with honey and crackers.

I was a bit of a culinary snob for a large portion of my life despite the semi-regular bouts of nausea and vomiting. When I lost the ability to eat food in my thirties, I lamented all the snacks I turned down over the years.

There was just something about eating in a medical setting that didn't do it for me, or at least, it didn't before I lost my ability to eat solid food.

But I eventually accepted food from one patient; he first came to see me to establish care for his annual biometric evaluation.

Biometric evaluations are tied to patients' health insurance premiums, and they need to meet quarterly goals to generate discounts. Patients could get points for completing a preventative exam that included a lipid panel and blood sugar check and they could get additional points for going to the dentist, getting eye exams, and the like. At the end of each quarter, your premium would reflect where you stood in the wellness program. Many patients took their frustrations directly out on me as a primary care provider, straight up blaming me for healthcare discrimination. While I sympathized, I was just a cog in the machine, and all I could do was log my findings.

You were either compliant or not.

When this patient came for his appointment, my nurse warned me he wouldn't give any straight answers. They were a thirty-five-year-old man with a relatively empty medical chart but two unassigned psychiatric medications. It was just one of those cases where you jump in and just see what happens once you're in the room. My nurse reassured me he didn't seem violent at all and so I went with it; they just seemed a little odd. I introduced myself and shared my background, and asked if they had any questions.

"Well, I don't, but the others might." He answered.

I narrowed my eyes but didn't probe.

We started at the beginning; I liked to go through each patient's health history to ensure it was correct and up to date. Patients would always get copies of their reports from me so that, no matter who they followed up with, they were in charge of their own accurate healthcare information.

"It says here you have no known allergies."

"I don't, but who knows."

"You should know," I quipped back with a tilt of my head to indicate amusement, not frustration.

That was the right tone to take because they cracked a sly smile and shrugged. They were on an antidepressant, and was requesting a refill of his benzodiazepine prescription. This is a controlled substance and, while it works well at calming anxiety attacks, it can be addictive, so should only be used as a rescue medication or a maintenance medication under the careful care of a psychiatrist.

Unfortunately, we live in America, and the state of mental healthcare is abysmal. Not everyone has access to a psychiatrist and often if they are lucky enough to access a primary care provider, that's where the care falls. Primary care providers are not psychiatric experts. They can often handle basic, garden-variety depression, but once things start going sideways into the worlds of delusions, paranoia, and suicidal ideation, they tend to peace out.

"Can you tell me the diagnosis associated with your antidepressant?"

"D.I.D." He crossed his arms over his chest and didn't elaborate.

"Well, that makes a whole lot more sense now!" I clapped.

"Wait, you know it?" It was his turn to be confused.

"I know it's not kosher to call it Multiple Personality Disorder anymore, but yeah, I know it. I'm interested to learn about your experiences."

"Ha! OK then!" He was pleasantly surprised by my reaction.

"How many personalities do you have and are they active?" I couldn't wait to listen.

And I listened. And listened. I think I spent at least an hour with him as they told me stories from different timelines. I will never understand clinicians that don't take every opportunity to learn about rare stories directly from the source. Over the years when I'd establish myself as a patient with a new primary care provider, I'd constantly be disappointed. Not only were they not familiar with Autoimmune Hepatitis as my historical diagnosis, but they also weren't curious. They never asked me questions. They just clicked the box that said hepatitis and asked me about IV drug use.

They consistently ignored my story.

So, I didn't mind that I got backed up that day while documenting after hours because this story was interesting. I knew the time I spent with them that day is why they chose to keep seeing me year after year, and why I was able to help when their personalities finally came out to play.

Formerly referred to as Multiple Personality Disorder, Dissociative Identity Disorder (D.I.D.) is a complex, chronic condition characterized by disruption in autobiographical memory and in the sense of having a unified identity. The disorder has been most commonly conceptualized as originating in the context of severe trauma during the patient's childhood. There was a small part of me that knew disassociating was never normal, despite the fact that I had been doing it ever since I could remember.

If you remember, my pediatricians reassured my parents I was normal.

But for other patients, disassociation is a big red flag. Disassociation is defined as a disruption of and/or discontinuity in the normal integration of consciousness, memory, identity, emotion, perception, body representation, motor control, and behavior. When one or more of these functions is disrupted, characteristic impairments can be seen and are broken up by deficits in the following four areas:

1. Consciousness:
   Decreased responsiveness to external stimuli.
2. Memory:
   Dissociative amnesia is a memory impairment in which the patient can no longer recall autobiographical information which is traumatic or stressful.
3. Identity:
   Confusion or discontinuation of who you are as a person.
4. Environment:
   Impaired connection to the patient's surroundings can include awareness of their body, self, and external environment.

Within these four parameters, patients may experience a variety of symptoms including amnesia, depersonalization, derealization, self-alteration, and trance-like states. If an individual does not endorse amnesia, they cannot be diagnosed with this condition. The presence of recurrent memory gaps is a requirement in the current DSM-5, and patients will typically report periods of time, sometimes up to hours or more, that they cannot remember. These periods may be associated with certain mood or behaviors and, over time, observers can start to determine a pattern in the personalities that present.

It wasn't until I got to graduate school that I realized I had been experiencing depersonalization and derealization my entire life. As a child and teenager, after a particularly bad episode of night terrors, it would take days, sometimes weeks, for me to feel like the world was normal. The only way I can describe it is that the world is slightly off kilter. It's like looking at a photograph through a foggy pane of glass, tipped just a few degrees off center. Eventually, I realized certain triggers would cause me to disassociate including certain turns of phrases but I didn't know that when I met this patient.

Depersonalization is defined as a feeling of detachment or estrangement from oneself or feeling like you are outside your own body. Derealization is the feeling that the external world is strange or unreal; you feel as if you are experiencing the world in a dreamlike state, and nothing is fixed.

It's extremely upsetting.

Self-alteration is the sense that one part of your body is markedly different from another part. This can manifest itself as a variety of body dysmorphia syndromes, alien limb syndrome, or D.I.D., but is not as common a presentation. Finally, trance-like states have been reported in the gross majority of D.I.D. patients. It is described as a narrowing of one's awareness of the immediate surroundings into stereotype behaviors or movements that are experienced as beyond one's control.

For example, rocking.

Rocking back and forth can be very soothing, it is one of my stimming behaviors, but it can also progress to self-harm very easily. How many of us have joked about the cliched psych patient rocking back and forth muttering to themselves in the corner?

How many of us have actually become that patient?

Well, until you have, approach them with an open mind and an even more open heart, because all humans are only a trauma away from disintegration.

But here's where it starts to get controversial: No one can agree why D.I.D. happens.

There are still clinicians who will dismiss psychiatric presentations because they don't understand them. They assume it must be "all in their heads" because there's not an easy mechanism of injury or clear pathology. It's a cascade of environmental stressors, genetic predispositions, and socioeconomic factors. Again, in medicine, if we don't understand the pathology behind a presentation, it will get dismissed, passed along, and bucked to the next person. Clinicians have horribly large egos, and it takes a lot to tell a patient that you simply "don't know" what is happening.

But honesty trumps ego every single time, in my book.

The trauma model of D.I.D. states patient presentations will feature personality states associated with specific, traumatic experiences. Classic examples include a patient reverting to a terrified, crying child or an angry authority figure. This patient had both male and female personalities ranging from five to fifty-three years old, but after years of intensive therapy, they all had reached an integrated state.

Some clinician researchers consider D.I.D. as more of a fragmentation of the identity and discontinuities in memory and identity experienced by the patient as intrusions. These intrusive thoughts can spur an overlapping, shifting, and interference between states of personality rather than a specific switch. When this patient first met me, they were fully integrated and had been for several years. They did this with intensive in and outpatient therapy, medication, and a strong support system.

This patient distanced himself from the early childhood traumas that triggered the original split. They were married, happily for a while, and had a young adult son that was close with him.

Over the years, we enjoyed an easy-going primary care relationship. I kept their cholesterol in check, and he'd make me smile with stories every visit. Their son was a military man, so it wasn't uncommon for them to bring treats back stateside, and one day the patient brought treats from Japan for me: Matcha Marshmallows

My eyes lit up as I saw the emerald green globes, and the plastic crinkled as I scooped them up.

"They're packaged so I figured you'd eat them." They smirked, knowing I never accepted food.

"What do they taste like?" I squished them through the plastic a little more, enjoying the sensation in my hands.

"A little citrusy and a little dry, if I'm being honest."

I opened the bag and plopped one in my mouth, letting the emerald sugar bump up my energy for another appointment. They were strangely dry and had a bit of a textural grain from the ground green tea. I closed the bag and told him I'd share the treats with my husband.

When I brought them home, my husband devoured them without hesitation. He asked which patient brought them and I simply told him one of my favorites. You can't really share your stories with family in medicine; it's considered a violation of patient privacy, and rightfully so, which is why all of these cases are fictionalized unless explicit permission was granted.

"They must be OK if you ate them. They're not crazy or anything, right?" He asked between mouthfuls of green goo.

"About as crazy as me," I quipped.

A few months after they gave me the candy, they made an appointment, and their demeanor was very different. They had bags under their eyes and their inner arms were scratched and sliced.

As we settled into the room I asked them, "Who am I talking to right now?"

"It's me. But. The others are here. And. And I'm having a hard time knowing when they came back." Their voice was quiet and halted. They didn't quite have a stutter, but I could see they were having a harder time communicating verbally.

"How long has this been happening?" I pointed to the horizontal cuts decorating their arm with concern in my voice.

"It's been a few weeks at least."

"What's changed since I last saw you?"

Suffice it to say, the stressors in his life became too much and triggered a relapse. From what we could deduce, two of his personalities had returned to respond to her external circumstances. One of his personalities was a teenage girl who was prone to smoking, chewing gum, and engaging in body mutilation. She was a defensive personality, and she came out when she felt threatened. The other personality was a harder, older, angrier man but I never found out exactly what happened to him because he left the state to seek care at an inpatient facility.

The teenager persona came out first, spitting, scratching, and screaming at their family when they were in control of the body. Like many teenage girls who feel an overwhelming lack of control about their life, this personality started taking out her frustrations and aggressions onto their inner arms. Each day the original patient would find a few more lacerations and mend them, praying no one at work wondered why they started wearing long sleeves in the summer.

I met her, the teenager, once, briefly, while we were speaking. She just wanted someone to listen.

I listened and I told her I wanted to help.

My patient wrestled the personality away and they all accepted my help.

When I finally fractured, I thought of them and their marshmallows, and I finally understood how someone could forget everything.

Autism Speaks for Itself

Looking back at the early education system of the American 90s, I can't help but be appalled at how we were treated. An entire generation of children went undiagnosed with a variety of neurodivergent presentations, and it's because we fell through the cracks. Thankfully, the way we talk about autism now is shifting dramatically to listening to the lived experiences of autistic people and it's about damn time.

Brown Eyes, as I took to calling him, was a six-year-old boy and he had no problem maintaining eye contact with me. I found myself growing fond of him because he was a curious person with wide brown eyes that would stare into mine with quiet contemplation. Even though he wasn't verbal, he could still communicate with me, and others, if only they paid enough attention.

His mother advocated fiercely for her son, and it was through her I first experienced the culture associated with Autism Speaks. I am not a fan of Autism Speaks. I truly believe their marketing campaigns are a large reason why neurodivergent adults struggle to claim their identities: they are marred with shame.

Autism Speaks was founded in 2005 by Bob Wright, vice chairman of General Electric, after his grandson was diagnosed with autism. They are widely regarded as a hateful organization by autistic autism advocates because the organization perpetuates the idea that autism is a disease as opposed to a neurotype. Autism Speaks once created a marketing campaign which insinuated that autism stole children away from their parents. They went so far to publish the following quote on their website and in various marketing campaigns:

"This disease has taken our children away. It's time to get them back."

Where did we go?

We were here all along, but instead of listening to the children in distress, they were placed into behavioral groups, given electro-shock therapy, or medicated into oblivion. Families are drawn to organizations like Autism Speaks because they create a culture in which the neurotypical family is surrounded by like-minded parents. This support, this community, is vital to many but when an organization infantilizes and excludes the very people they are supposed to help, I have a problem. Autism Speaks enforces this culture of infantilization and propagates a narrative that having an autistic child is a tragedy. I grew up with Autism Speaks in the background and so whenever I would wonder about my anxieties and sensory processing issues, I would simply dismiss autism as an option.

I didn't look like those boys. I didn't act like those boys. I didn't want to be a tragedy.

The night I realized I was masking more than just garden-variety depression and anxiety was the night I went to a stadium concert with a few friends after work.

Brown Eyes was the last patient of the day and we were following up on some eating issues he had. He was sitting on the floor and I was sitting on one of the chairs facing his mother, pretty uncomfortably, if I was being honest. I can't sit normally; I prefer to sit cross-legged at all times. Brown Eyes was rocking slightly and had a blue glove-balloon in his hand. He was clearly stimming and enjoying the bouncing sensation of the balloon on his leg. Truth be told, I was more interested in his balloon than I was in listening to Autism Mom debate whether or not she should force him to eat more vegetables.

(The answer is no.)

He hated the texture of fresh fruit or veggies and would spit them out or throw them forcefully around the room. Looking at him while considering the problem, I slid myself onto the floor and continued chatting with his mother unbroken, but now my physical body was parallel to Brown Eyes.

He threw his hands forward, flinging the balloon into the center of the room and I understood it was an invitation to play. His mother didn't want to play so she redirected him by giving him the balloon back. He immediately threw it forward. Before she could intercept the balloon or tell him to "behave" again, I reached forward and I tapped it back at him.

He tapped it back to me.

We continued playing with the makeshift balloon for at least another five minutes all while I continued to carry a conversation with Autism Mom in which I suggested that perhaps forcing him to eat anything fresh was the problem. Perhaps she should work with him to avoid textures he didn't like. We arrived at a conclusion:

Freeze dried fruit and veggies.

The crispy, crunchy, sweet and salty snacks could be perfectly reproduced each time without any weird squishy, wet, squelchy, flavors that were unexpected. I didn't know it at the time, but my suggestion that afternoon transformed Brown Eyes' diet literally overnight. It was as simple as working with him instead of forcing him to comply. I knew so many of his family concerns were based on how normal he "looked" and "acted". For me, I was more concerned about elevating his glimmers and minimizing his triggers, but I could only recommend so much before I isolated a parent.

It's always such a fine line.

I left the clinic conflicted, but I was happy to have given his mother a plan that wasn't based on Applied Behavioral Analysis or stress habituation. I kept thinking about how my parents supported me during times of high anxiety as opposed to forcing me into a situation I couldn't handle and I was grateful. I too understood the anxiety, fear, and frustration of biting into something you expected to be sweet and firm only to have a mouthful of sour mush seep out.

I met up with my friends and we all went onward to the stadium to shake our groove thangs. And shake them we did, but I was not without my consequences.

As I approached the stadium, I immediately felt a wave of panic wash over me as the crowds turned into marching ants; too many too count. We joined the din of eager concert goers and we found ourselves close to the stage some forty rows away from the man making the music of the night. My friends sat, and danced, to my left, but strangers boxed me in on all other sides. The smell of sweat pierced my nostrils and burned a hole in the back of my head and, when the bass started to swell, I felt like I was going to swoon in the worst of ways.

I followed their lead and danced along to the music but I realized quickly that I wasn't having the same kind of fun that they were. I enjoyed this band in the comfort of my home, but turned up with speakers in a stadium, I simply couldn't cope.

That night, I had more nightmares.

The next day, I started Googling "Autism in Women," and what I found was startling mostly because I realized women were completely excluded from the development of diagnostic criteria. Further, we had no concrete examples of what healthy, thriving adult autistics looked like and so I found myself falling down a timeline rabbit hole of neurodiversity.

Autism was introduced originally as a symptom of schizophrenia around the turn of the 20th century in 1908 when German psychiatrist Eugene Bleuler first used the term. He described autism as a retreat into an inner life, or sanctum, to avoid facing the harshness of reality. Originally considered purely a psychological problem, we know now that autism is a mixture of biological and environmental factors, not entirely understood.

For decades, though, autism was considered to be a psychological disorder of childhood. Dr. Leo Kanner, a child psychiatrist at Johns Hopkins University School of Medicine, identified early infantile autism in 1943. He asserted that this unique condition was characterized by obsessiveness, deficits in social behavior, and a need for sameness in routine. Children identified with early infantile autism tended to dislike disruptions in their routines.

Only a year later, across the ocean, Dr. Hans Asperger, a pediatrician at the University of Vienna, expanded on the field of autism by coining the phrase "autistic psychopathy." His area of interest, as one might guess, was the high-functioning autistics, and it was his namesake that was used to describe "high-functioning individuals who showed social deficits." These were the weird kids. The children who could be put to work, instead of institutionalized, were diagnosed with Aspergers. They were the ones who weren't "quite right" but nothing was obviously wrong with them and Dr. Asperger argued that their skills could be quite beneficial if utilized. This 'otherness' would become a recurring theme in the diagnostic workup of autistic children.

Back in the United States, in 1967, Kanner published a theory that Refrigerator Mothers were responsible for autism in their children. He postulated that cold, uncaring mothers who did not nurture their children were responsible for traumatizing their offspring and therefore creating autism as a response. They were cold like refrigerators, he argued, and that's why the children were similarly cold to social interactions. There was no equivalent term for cold, uncaring fathers.

Blaming the Refrigerator Mothers was further championed by Bruno Bettelheim, and together with Kanner the two men convinced a generation of mothers that it was their emotionally cold and distant parenting that caused mental distress in the kiddos. This held water until the 1970s when a study conducted by Susan

Folstein and Michael Rutter found that autism was more common in identical twins but not so if the twins were fraternal. This suggested a genetic link and paved the way for the condition to be taken more seriously and less psychosomatically.

Six years before I was born, in 1980, the Diagnostic and Statistical Manual of Mental Disorders included autism as a unique entity. It was recognized as a developmental disorder, separate from schizophrenia, and all previous requirements of hallucinations were removed from the diagnostic criteria. Autism was broken down into four subtypes for pediatricians to diagnose:

1. Infantile Autism
2. Residual Autism
3. Childhood-Onset Pervasive Developmental Disorder
4. Atypical Autism

A year after I was born, in 1987, the DSM-III was modified to broaden the concept of autism to include milder symptoms. This was also the same year that Ivar Lovaas, widely considered the pioneer of Applied Behavioral Analysis, published a study showing improvement in symptoms of autistic children after intensive behavioral therapy.

Except those that survived intense behavioral therapy report a very different experience.

It hurt. A lot.

And it definitely didn't help. Applied Behavioral Analysis is little more than dog training using positive and negative reinforcement to convince autistic children to "act like their peers". The problem with this is that autistic individuals do not need to act more like their peers, they need to be given the space and accommodations to be themselves.

The general American public wasn't aware of autism until it was popularized by the media. Medical media is how many of us learn about health and so, when Dustin Hoffman hit the silver screen as Raymond Babbitt in the 1988 movie "Rain Man," he was seen as an example of autism. While Mr. Babbitt's portrayal is based on a true story, it only shows one experience and cannot possibly encapsulate all individuals on the spectrum. Yet it created that awareness in the zeitgeist. At the same time, it also created an indelible stereotype that pegs autistics as idiot savants with little representation elsewhere in the media to balance those potentially harmful assumptions.

The Babbitt story is important but it sure would have been a lot more helpful if at the same time positive representations were depicted. It wasn't until the story of Temple Grandin came out that I saw a female representation of autism in adulthood, and I started to feel like I wasn't just a weirdo.

Mary Temple Grandin was born on August 29th, 1947, and is perhaps one of the most famous Animal Behaviorists in the world. When she was born, she was diagnosed with "brain damage," but this was later debunked by cerebral imaging conducted in 2010 at the University of Utah. She is one of the first autistic people to document her lived experience and is considered to be an authority on livestock. She is able to visualize the world much in the same way the animals she studies do: She sees patterns other people don't.

In her case, she was lucky to have a mother who advocated for her care. At the time of her diagnosis in the early 1950s, the standing recommendation for any autistic-appearing individuals was lifelong institutionalization. While her father agreed with the doctors, her mother fought tooth and nail and ensured she was surrounded by affirming and supportive caregivers, educators, and family members. Temple's mother effectively obliterated the Refrigerator Mother myth by demonstrating fierce advocacy for her child. Now Temple has published over sixty scientific papers and is a faculty member of Animal Sciences in the College of Agricultural Sciences at Colorado State University.

In 2013, three years after I started practicing medicine, she published The Autistic Brain: Thinking Across the Spectrum, in which she details the three different types of thinking experienced by autistics:

Visual Thinkers (like Grandin) think in photographically specific images.

Musical/Mathematical Thinkers (like Babbitt) think in patterns and are often adept at programming.

Verbal Logic Thinkers (like me) think in word details and are hyperlexic, often gravitating toward languages and history.

Rather than try to explain autism as a pathology or an offshoot of schizophrenia, Temple taught that autism is just another way of experiencing the world. Much of the "bad behavior" associated with autism is present when individuals are in distress and, when accommodations are made for sensory differences, much of the pathology dissipates. First, her mother asked what would happen if her daughter was supported instead of isolated, and then Grandin continued that crusade herself.

The United States Congress passed legislation in 1990 to include autism as a category of educational disability, opening up, theoretically, resources in school settings. The DSM-IV was updated to include Aspergers as a separate subcategory in 1994, but progress was dashed in 1998 when the former doctor, Andrew Wakefield, published a report in the Lancet suggesting that the Measles, Mumps, and Rubella vaccine may predispose children to autism. While this study only included twelve children and had no controls, it received widespread media attention resulting in a decline in vaccinations and the development of anti-vax "autism parents."

Even though he lost his medical license, and even though thimerosal, a mercury-based preservative used in vaccines, was removed from childhood vaccines in 2001, the damage was irrevocable.

I continued researching autism and I finally stumbled upon a 2002 study conducted by the Center of Disease Control which indicated that 1 in every 150 children in the United States had autism. Twelve years later, in 2014, the CDC would update their numbers to reflect 1 in every 59 children screened had autism. I had read enough to know that, if I were being honest with myself, I had a lot in common with Temple, Babbitt, and Brown Eyes.

My husband was skeptical. My mother was skeptical. My best friend was skeptical. But the more I read, the more I realized I was autistic. I started combing my memory for instances in which I misinterpreted what someone was saying and I realized I couldn't come up with an example, but not because there weren't enough examples. There were too many. I couldn't think of a time when I *didn't* struggle with understanding what people were saying.

In grade school, I latched onto a series of rotating girls because I thought that's what I was supposed to do. I thought, if I imitated the popular kids long enough, I would be just like them. My only real friend from grade school was a quirky young boy who also peered at his peers from behind well-worn Goosebumps covers. He was the only person I would share my treasured books with, and he didn't make fun of me the way the girls did. We both preferred to get lost in literary worlds. We'd read next to each other, not speaking, in what I only realized was parallel play years later.

In middle school, I hung around the goth, theater, and emo kids, but I never felt entirely included. If I didn't specifically get an invitation, I was not invited. Obviously.

I've since learned that's not always the case.

As an adult, I prepared for an evaluation with a neuropsychiatrist that specialized in Adult Autism. I compiled my symptoms as if I were preparing to defend myself in court. I looked at the diagnostic criteria set forth by the current DSM and I wondered if this was going to be the first time I was honest with a doctor since childhood. I had long since wondered about the vivid nightmares, the lingering sensory dysfunctions, and the mounting anxieties, but as I pursued school, I neglected my original patient: myself.

I had not seen a cardiologist since high school. I had not seen my gastroenterologist since they discontinued the chemotherapy. I had seen a therapist on and off but I found myself doubting his intelligence and his recommendations when he kept circling back to suggestions that I exercise more and get fresh air. I was an oxymoron: I went into medicine to save myself, but I never gave anyone an accurate history.

So, I set down to write an accurate history of my mental and emotional symptoms. When I was done, I looked at the list and felt ashamed. The words felt like accusations.

Socks. Sand on my feet. Skin to skin contact. Wolf Club. Friendship group. Panic attacks. Clothing tags. Zippers. Fucking zippers. Glare. Headaches. Mayonnaise. Bass. Tapping. Rocking. Singing.

It all started with socks.

Being unable to tolerate certain textures on my feet was a recurring theme during my early childhood. Even now as an adult, at the time of this writing I only own three pairs of socks I actually tolerate wearing. I truly detest the sensation of socks on my feet but I can't handle being barefoot either. When I was a toddler, I had such an epic fit on an airplane over not wanting to wear socks, I ended up repeatedly hitting myself and subsequently kicking the woman's seat in front of me.

In hindsight, I was repetitiously beating my legs until the trigger was alleviated because I was overwhelmed with the pain of sensory overload.

If I looked even further back into my childhood, I was brought back to memories of meltdowning on the beach. I would leave the solace of the water only to have my feet dotted with billions of shards of sand, immediately sending me into a sensory overload that drove me back into the water. My mother would beckon me back out, but as soon as my feet hit the sand again, the cycle repeated and, if I couldn't wash my extremities off, I became extremely distressed.

I also hated the touch of my sister's skin as a small child. As for my sister, I avoided holding her hand or touching her face because her skin was simply too soft, so holding it made me uncomfortable. I once tried to explain that her touch caused me physical discomfort, but I was little, and my tongue was clumsy.

She cried.

I hurt her, so very badly, so many times, and I didn't even understand it.

My inability to connect with children my own age stood out like a sore thumb. I would engage with children, and I loved to play pretend as a wolf, but as everyone else aged out of that type of childish play, I found myself wondering which script to flip into to keep passing.

As I struggled with making friends, I was placed in an Applied Behavioral Analysis program. Once a week, I'd join a group of children who had a variety of behavioral issues though no clear diagnoses. I remember the program in bits and flashes. I remember there was a dark room that always seemed to glow with VHS instructional videos. The television that beamed these images of smiling children at us was ancient in the way of outdated technology, but the message was as old as time:

Conform or get the fuck out.

These videos theoretically "taught" us how to approach a group of children to start playing with them. They had us role play how to start and maintain friendships within the group. Unfortunately, I was occasionally paired with a student with roaming hands and I hated how often he would try to touch me or play with my hair.

His hands would slither over to my seat, grabbing clothing or my braid, and I'd yelp, growling at him, "Leave me alone!"

"Katie, we don't yell," the Facilitator counselor admonished me.

"But he won't stop!" I complained.

"And what do we say when we don't want to play with someone?" she asked in a sing-song voice.

The moment the Facilitator turned her attention back to the television, the room darkened and flickering, he would start touching me again. He wasn't the only one who was touching me inappropriately, but it wasn't until years later when a teacher put out an anonymous box did I get the help I so desperately needed as a vulnerable child. I waited until no one was around and I scribbled the question that prompted the teacher to step in, finally:

What do you do if someone keeps touching you and won't stop no matter what you do?

You ask for help. In my experience though, it wasn't until I wrote the request for help down that something happened about it.

Autistic people are at risk for emotional, physical, and sexual abuse. I hung my head as I compared my early childhood relationships to high school and beyond. I reflected upon the highly dysfunctional trysts I had with various boys in college, and I realized each and every time I was not an entirely cognizant participant. I misinterpreted so many cues I just can't count them.

Considering my social relationships in graduate school, I realized how bitterly I fought with my peers over having the curtains open in class during sunny days. I argued that the intense glare kept me from seeing my laptop screen and gave me a wicked headache. Only two other participants in the class of forty agreed with me, but, ultimately, I got my way at the expense of the camaraderie of my peers.

Driving into the appointment with the neuropsychiatrist, I felt my heart in my chest as I waited to meet with her. My story tumbled out and, to my great surprise, at the end of our first session (which was two hours long after a nurse intake), she reassured me that I wasn't crazy.

"You certainly show signs of autism," she confirmed, "but you also have significant childhood and medical trauma we need to unpack."

"So, you think I might be on the spectrum?" There was a part of me that felt dirty saying it out loud, that I was just looking for problems where there weren't any and seeking attention.

I know now that a large part of that had to do with the gendered diagnosis structure and the malignant portrayals by organizations such as Autism Speaks. Deconstructing internalized ableism is difficult but necessary because we deserve not only to survive but to thrive.

"Yes, I do. We'll continue this next session." She stood up and I knew it was time to go.

On the way out, her receptionist warned me the waitlist for her was long and, while I was now an established patient, her next appointment was in four weeks. I eagerly took the spot, tears in my eyes behind my sunglasses because I thought we'd start uncovering the roots of my parasomnias and neuroses, and I could finally start understanding the pieces that were missing.

Three weeks later, I got a letter in the mail saying she was no longer practicing medicine.

I was devastated.

I was offered an appointment with her replacement. He was not a neuropsychiatrist. He spent our entire follow-up session reading my chart out loud to me, and it was clear he didn't have the expertise to continue our evaluation. I put my mental health back on the shelf, along with my physical health, because, like so many other patients, I had hit another dead end.

You Saved My Child

I never wanted children of my own, which is probably a good thing because I always assumed because of my medical conditions, it was off the table. I do have a great bedside manner with children, though, and I've always been mistaken for a pediatrician in my practice. I don't claim to be a pediatrician. In fact, I've been known to snort loudly when I'm mistaken for one.

What I am, however, is someone who understands how to talk to children.

Kids don't communicate the way adults do; everything they do is natural until adults impose order. Consider, we tend to beat communication into children over the years so that they are mimicking what we already do, but that doesn't always work. The apraxic child who is unable to physically move the muscles of their lips, tongue, and jaw may be better served with a combination of sign language and written expression. The autistic child may not be able to tolerate an examination with bare skin-on-skin contact but might be perfectly comfortable with the texture of nitrile-gloved hands and will respond if you model the behavior on a parent first. It's all about figuring out the 'how' and 'why' behind why a child acts the way they do, and then you can start to communicate with them on their level.

It can be as simple as getting on the ground with them, like with Brown Eyes.

When I enter a room, if the child is crying, I might ignore them completely or I might cry back at them. This approach works best in a toddler-aged kiddo because it shocks them out of their tantrum. Sometimes. If it doesn't work, I'll continue to talk to the parents until the child is ready to interact with me.

Kids are also plain weird and do strange things which is why some of my best stories come from my time in pediatrics. I started to take a liking to adolescent medicine, and this blossomed the more time I spent in Primary Care.

One day, our receptionist got a panicked phone call from a parent who informed us her child had a plastic bead stuck in her ear. The child and I had a great relationship, so she was a willing participant in the procedure. When we first met, she was enthralled by my waist-length golden tresses. The Disney adaptation of Rapunzel had only just come out and my then-boyfriend had more than a passing resemblance to Flynn Rider, so it only made logical sense that I was not Kateland, I was Doctor Tangled.

"Hi Doctor Tangled!" The child chirped proudly when her mom brought her into the pediatric room.

"Hey, you. I understand you got a bead in your year. How'd that happen?"

"Not a bead!" She made a scrunched-up face, clarifying exaggeratedly. "A ball."

The mother and I looked at each other, "A ball?"

Remember how I said kids are weird and it's all about figuring out how they see the world? In my early days, I'd ask children if I could look in their ears to see what was in there. The last time I saw her, I used that technique to check her ears. I told her there were two monkeys, one in each ear and that was my great mistake.

"I wanted to give the monkeys a ball to play with." She smiled.

And sure enough, there was a glittering, plastic, blue bead jammed right up against her eardrum, and it was pretty snug. I couldn't get forceps around it for a manual removal so I decided to get creative. Getting creative is one of my favorite phrases because you don't always have all the tools you need in rural medicine and it's good practice to be flexible in your approach.

I broke out the DermaBond and an ear curette. DermaBond is a surgical glue that parents praise, because it allows us to close lacerations without so much as a pin prick. It dries rather quickly, so I thought I could put a few drops of the DermaBond on the end of the plastic ear scoop, hold it against the bead, and pull it out. Thankfully, the bead did exactly as I predicted and, twenty minutes later, we were foreign body free.

Peeking at her eardrum once more, I informed her the monkeys had moved out for good.

"What? Why?" Her eyes flickered in concern.

"I should have told you this at your kindergarten check, but I forgot. When you become a big girl and go to school, the monkeys move out."

"Oh." She chewed on that for a second and then hopped up to play, "OK."

Kid logic works best for kids. Adult logic only occasionally works on adults.

As I built my primary care practice, I started seeing recurrent needs with the children. They were almost all overweight, if not clinically obese, and more than a few were starting to demonstrate signs of diabetes, hypertension, and high cholesterol. I wasn't certain how to proceed with metabolic syndrome in a twelve-year-old girl when my medical training taught me that was a condition for middle-aged men with a penchant for beers and wings.

Meanwhile, a variety of weight loss reality competitions were taking the country by storm.

People were tuning in from all over to watch obese individuals compete to lose the pounds on primetime television. It was not safe. It was a horrible example of reality television sensationalizing medical conditions, but when our primary care office wanted to host a series of weight loss competitions, I was the point person.

I loved creating community programming and received several awards for my work during my time in primary care. I was given no direction by our management team, so I started small by drafting up nutritional posters for snacks in the breakroom in English and Spanish. This was well received and so I then got permission to start a Zumba with clinic staff class. Every Saturday, I'd get to the clinic an hour and a half early, and I'd exercise with my patients.

It was a "put your money where your mouth is" sort of situation.

I'd often recommend exercise to my patients, to which they'd complain they never have the time, and then I'd invite them to a

Saturday session. It became one of my more popular programs and I'll never forget seeing the one sixty-something-year-old man shaking his booty with the thirty-year-old Hispanic mammas. The nutritional posters and exercise class went well, but it was the weight loss competitions that our clinic sponsored that left a bad taste in my mouth. Adults could opt in for a weight loss challenge and at the end of two quarters whichever man and woman lost the most got a monetary prize.

It got nasty.

Who knew adults would get so vindictive over their coworkers' weight losses? I found myself abandoning the program after the participants fought over the prizes and after I realized multiple participants got triggered into disordered eating. After two years of running these adult based programs, I wanted to focus on prevention rather than stimulating competition. At the time, I was an active CrossFit participant, even training under a few World Champions, so I pitched a "CrossFit for Kids Summer Camp" to replace my adult programming.

Partnering with a local gym, I created a program in which twelve kids were sent to six weeks of summer camp where they learned the foundations of body movements. I didn't want my program to be focused on numbers and calories, knowing how much that affected me as a child and then watching the grown adults act as fools with my weight loss competitions. I wanted to empower these children with functional goals and try to prevent them from picking up on the unhealthy habits of the adults around them.

At the start of both summers, the children would get a bio-metric screening which included height, weight, cholesterol, and blood sugar, and they would be asked to set a functional physical goal. This could be as simple as running a mile (or walking it), or it could be finally completing a pull up! Each kid had to come up with something different that wasn't based around a number on a scale.

At the end of the program, to celebrate, I threw them a giant picnic complete with Subway catering (gotta keep those meals fresh!) and a water balloon fight. Unlike the other staff members, AKA the adults in the room, I was all about the water balloon fight. I didn't sit back in my white coat; I was throwing neon-colored blobs with the youngest of them and I was relishing every minute.

For a moment, we weren't worrying about scales or sizes; we were simply reveling in what it meant to be human. We were en-joying sunshine, green grass, and time with friends. We were moving in purposeful ways and enriching each other's lives. We were, in a word, free for just a moment.

You never know the impact you make on a person until they tell you.

At this point in my career, it was time for a change and my husband and I were preparing to move to Vermont to be closer to family on the East coast. Before I left my clinic to travel cross-country to start my career in Urgent Medicine, one of my former Primary Care patients thanked me in a way I wasn't expecting. This young man, when we first met years earlier, struggled with social engagements, and I was treating him for early high blood

pressure, elevated sugar, and cholesterol, which was a scary proposition at any age.

"Thank you for saving my life." He looked me directly in the
eyes.

"Aw, you're welcome," I started to blush and tried to stop him,
but he pushed forward.

"No, really."

And then he admitted when he first met me as a teenager, he
was thinking about ending it all.

Shocked, I looked at the young man in front of me. Not once
did he mention he was suicidal, and I cursed myself for missing
it.

How did I miss it?

He promised me he would keep up the healthy lifestyle and
keep in touch over the years, but, the sands of time wait for no
one and I never heard from him again. After killing Bobby so
many years prior, I felt some small sliver of redemption because,
if I could save one suicidal teenager and help him grow up into a
man, maybe there was still hope for me yet.

Life Before a Diagnosis

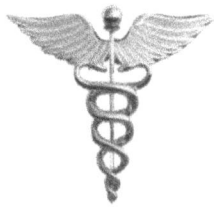

It's Just a Rash

It was cancer.

It was unmistakable.

It had to be cancer.

There was no other explanation as I stared at my pale face in the mirror, wiping sour vomit from my chin. My health had taken an unusual turn since moving to Vermont. My worst nightmare was cancer catching up to me in my thirties, a delayed side effect from my teenage regimen of oral immunosuppressants. Since arriving in the Green Mountain State, I'd wake up each morning with my stomach seized in pain, cramping and nausea giving way to severe diarrhea and vomiting. The pain reminded me of the liver lightning of my youth, but there was another layer to it. It was deeper and broader, and it was becoming more consistent. Unfortunately, no one in Vermont seemed to know what was happening to me and truthfully, neither did I.

I left Utah to be closer to my East coast family. It was a move made out of desperation and the hope that being closer to my family would alleviate the growing anxieties and neuroses that were plaguing my life and my relationships. By the time I left the Intermountain West, I had ballooned up to 222 lbs., using food as a primary source of comfort even as I taught children and adults how to lose weight without engaging in disordered eating. It was irony at its finest. As my weight increased, though, I started to notice a curious phenomenon:

I kept moving my car seat backwards.

More specifically, I kept adjusting the angle of the car so it went from keeping me in a relatively upright posture, to a reclined one. I couldn't sit up straight because, when I did, my stomach pain worsened. I blamed it on being fat, and so did my doctors.

I was in this position the morning I lost control of my car just an exit before my urgent care in Vermont. I found myself without any power to my steering column and, in my panic, I jerked the wheel frantically side by side. Like much of my life, I had absolutely no control over what came next. Suddenly, I was airborne, flying at seventy-five miles an hour toward the center ditch of a rural highway. The last thing I remember is being suspended in the crystalline air with the icy snowflakes dancing just outside the windows, my hot cup of coffee floating beside my face, and a voice drifted through my consciousness:

I guess this is happening now.

Instinctively, I went slack. Then everything was black.

But only for a moment, I think. It's hard to tell because the next thing I knew, a frantic couple was knocking at my window, trying to wake me up.

"Are you alive?" A woman yelled through the cold glass.

I nodded, my head fuzzy and full of snow. "Yes, I, I'm OK. I'm. I'm fine."

"No, you're not! We saw you fly! 911 is on the way!" She tried to open my door, but it was jammed. The metal was crunched beyond her capabilities.

I felt wet and, for a moment, I froze, thinking I urinated during my accident. But to my relief it was only the coffee and creamer. When the ambulance arrived, it took some time to get me out. I don't remember it all, but I was later told I was so anxious about my employer being mad at me for being late, I went so far as to call and text the manager while EMS was trying to free me. She was a young girl, without any experience in medicine, but she had a reputation for being an enforcer for our corporate overlords, so I didn't expect much sympathy for being late.

I babbled as I apologized for my tardiness and told her I'd be in as soon as they got me out of my car. It was only when she was informed by EMS staff that I was being transported to the hospital that my work let go of the idea of me coming in for that shift.

A head and neck CT cleared me to go home, but I would never be the same.

I suffered a concussion and bruising along my chest and abdomen where the seatbelt cut into my body. Despite my physical injuries, I was granted no reprieve from twelve-hour clinic shifts in front of screens performing high-level intellectual work. Immediately after the impact, I noticed my words left me for a while. The word loss and memory impairments from the crash improved over the next six months or so, but my health declined drastically in other ways. The nausea of my youth returned along with a dull, constant ache in my right shoulder that pierced into my right upper quadrant:

Liver, Lung, Gallbladder, Stomach…

The clinician in me chanted body parts like a mantra hoping to find an underlying pathology, but my primary care provider dismissed my concerns and claimed my bloodwork and scans were completely normal.

But it wasn't normal and suddenly, in addition to the brain fog, worsening abdominal pain, and heartburn with vomiting, I started rapidly losing weight. I wasn't trying to lose weight but it started falling off just the same.

Being a self-sufficient clinician in a state with atrocious healthcare, I decided to be proactive, and I started journaling my symptoms while implicating lifestyle changes. I cut out the rare alcohol I enjoyed and stayed away from citrus, spicy foods (not a problem for me), and anything too acidic. I choked down calcium carbonate, hating every minute of the chalky texture as it coated my lips. It wasn't enough, so I attempted a trial of omeprazole, a proton pump inhibitor, over the counter.

Then I started waking up with vomit in the back of my throat.

Then I couldn't hold my food down.

It got to the point where I couldn't even hold down a few bits of macaroni and cheese without vomiting profusely. My primary care provider had no problem suggesting another follow-up every three to six months to see how "lifestyle interventions went," which is code for diet and exercise. She suggested on multiple occasions that, while it was unfortunate I had heartburn, I should see the silver lining:

I was obese and I was losing weight! Hooray!

I kept practicing medicine and I kept wasting away.

While she didn't refer me despite my requests, she did saddle me with a monster of a placeholder diagnosis: gastroparesis. Gastroparesis is a symptom, not a diagnosis, and there is an ongoing patient advocacy campaign to increase funding for research. It is an umbrella term for decreased function, or motility, of the esophagus, stomach, intestines, and colon. In my case, it wasn't just heartburn I was experiencing, but the progressive loss of the ability to eat solid food.

I became the living dead, a zombie rotting from the inside out.

I went from gorging on gourmet meals to retching over a toilet bowl when I attempted anything more substantial than a cracker. I was desperate for answers and not just more pills to Band-Aid symptoms. Unfortunately, Band-Aids were all that the primary care office could offer me. They initially ruled out diabetes, hypothyroidism, and a bacterial infection of the stomach called Helicobacter Pylori, but that's where my doctor stopped her workup. She gave up and transferred my care to a local gastroenterologist.

Suddenly, I was under 150 pounds and I felt weak but thankfully the local gastroenterologist agreed we needed to do more tests. He started with a barium swallow at our local hospital. These swallows are a particular type of hell when you can't hold down your cookies because you are expected to drink a large quantity of this chalky liquid substance which then makes its way through your gastrointestinal system. A radiologist takes X-rays of the junk as it journeys outward, identifying any structural abnormalities along the way.

As an autistic woman, I knew I was going to struggle with the sensory overload of the terrible taste. The technician strapped me to the examination table, which was prepared to tilt this way and that to fully coat my innards. The radiologist offered me a brimming cup filled with white barium. I asked for my purse, noting I brought my own straw.

"It's too thick to drink with a straw." He stopped the nurse from getting my bag.

"Which is why I brought my own. May I please have my bag?" I repeated my request levelly.

Barium is too thick to suck up with a regular straw, but a Boba tea straw with its increased diameter provided me with an excellent way to force the liquid past my tongue. At least a little; even as I write this now, I gag recalling the way I felt suspended in that room.

When a patient requests an accommodation, attempts should be made to make it if it is reasonable. I had the foresight to recognize my sensory issues with taste and texture would make the test challenging if not outright painful for me, so I brought a straw to alleviate that overload. The physician shouldn't have questioned me but rather worked with me to minimize my pain.

Accessibility isn't just about ramps; it's about making medicine and life work for everyone.

The test revealed a hiatal hernia, an outpouching of my stomach through my diaphragm, prompting a referral off to a General Surgeon. Unfortunately, in Vermont, that meant a wait list of several months and the date just kept getting pushed back. It was when the general surgeon's receptionist called to reschedule yet again, this time during my gastric emptying study – a disgusting test in which you force a gastroparesis patient to eat radioactive eggs and take pictures – that a nurse found me sobbing hysterically in my room.

I couldn't stop crying, no matter what she said. Finally, I wrote on a piece of paper:

They just rescheduled me again with the surgeon. I'm sorry, I don't mean to be this hysterical. I'm just so tired of being in pain.

She hugged me and, even though I generally do not like to be touched, I hugged her back.

I was still seeing patients but no one knew how much pain I was in. I was hiding the fact I couldn't eat anymore by drinking lattes with whole milk on shift and sneaking sips of Boost. By the time I finished an outpatient urgent care shift, I was ready to collapse to the point where my husband started driving me to and from work.

I couldn't eat.

I couldn't drive.

I couldn't ride my bike.

I couldn't even have sex because the pain was overwhelming.

I couldn't figure out what was wrong with me and it felt like my world kept getting smaller.

That's something no one ever really talks about: how chronic illness makes your world small. Pain and disability can form you into something you never expected and, for me, I became an angry, bitter, tired person who lashed out at my husband and family whenever I was off work. I became reliant on the scripts I had developed over the years just to get through my clinic days, but whenever I went off script and tried to speak freely at home, it just came out as frustrated, misdirected anger.

At this point, I had switched to a different primary care provider who listened to my concerns more so than the first provider or my current gastroenterologist. She was the one that suggested I incorporate medical cannabis into my regimen because I couldn't tolerate oral pain medications without vomiting them up instantly.

At first, I struggled deeply with the introduction of cannabis into my regimen. That, to me, proved my mystery disease was cancer. Only cancer patients got weed, after all. Objectively, I knew that wasn't true and I had seen the effects it had for my husband firsthand, as he lives with Scheuermann's Disease. This is a type of progressive kyphosis, or hunch backing, which results in severe deformity and disability. His physicians offered him no solutions but plenty of narcotics over the years and he, having watched family and friends struggle with addiction, wanted no part of those prescriptions.

Nevertheless, each time I picked up my medication from the dispensary, I felt guilt and shame. It was a rescue medication, but it still carried such significant stigma that I labeled myself an addict simply for touching the stuff. In my mind, I bought into the idea that weed was only for addicts and the dying.

The medical bills were mounting so I kept clocking in day after day; I poured all my energy into my new practice and serving the patients who were also stuck in this healthcare desert with me. We all just wanted someone to listen to us. I kept struggling to put on a happy face while at work, but my rising medical costs, and the sinking realization that corporate urgent care is production medicine, where patients are lined up, evaluated, and discharged much like an assembly line, left me depressed. We were in the business of seeing as many patients as possible and production goals meant we were encouraged to see more than five patients per hour to be profitable.

Either way, I vowed to my staff at those rural clinics to do the best I could with what I had. I tried to ignore my growing frustrations with my employer and focus on the people in front of me instead of on my pain.

So, on the day I saw a pediatric patient the color of parchment, I knew it was cancer.

It was unmistakable.

There was no other explanation as I stared at the pale child in front of me. The clinic door closed with a click and the room felt chilly. She was one of my last patients of the day and her mother was desperate for a second opinion, according to my receptionist.

The kid's chart read "rash x 2 d," which told me that he was dealing with a skin eruption for the past 48 hours, but this kid looked chronic.

She wasn't just pale; it was translucent like the paper we used to line the exam tables. It was like looking at a ghost of a child except this four-year-old was very much flesh and blood, and she was in my urgent care. She was draped across her mother's lap, half asleep with nearly blue-lidded eyes from the veins pulsing softly.

"What brings you in today, Mom?"

"It's just a rash."

It's cancer, my mind screamed at me while I focused on her words so I wouldn't miss anything.

She shared how her child started getting these little red dots all over her lower legs two days ago. They hadn't been out in the woods or tall grass recently, no new detergents, and no one else in the household had similar symptoms. Her mother did endorse significant fatigue for the past six months, really since she had turned four, which the pediatrician repeatedly dismissed as normal. It was when she endorsed a history of fevers, and more specifically three febrile seizures without any documented temperature above 99 degrees, that I grew suspicious.

I looked at the child with pity in my eyes. I asked her if she could hop up on the table. She shook her head weakly; her mother gently placed her on the exam table and hiked up her pants to reveal a petechial rash going up her ankles to the mid-shins. The red capillary dots contrasted sharply with her parchment-colored skin and, when I pressed down firmly, they didn't blanch, which is to say, the red remained.

Her conjunctivas were pale, and her fingertips remained white when I pressed down on them, when a normal capillary refill response would be to pink right back up in under three seconds. She was beyond fatigued.

She was a ghost.

"Mom, I don't want to scare you, but I want to call her pediatrician. I'm very concerned this rash could be something more serious and I want to get some bloodwork."

"You can't do it here?" Disappointment flickered across her eyes, and I felt a stab of inadequacy.

"I don't have the capability to get what we need in this setting. She needs to be in a hospital."

Sometimes you just know.

This child reminded me so very much of Bobby and my time in oncology, I almost cried as I closed the door on her to go back to our nurse's station. It was fifteen minutes to five, which meant it was hit or miss if the pediatrician would even answer their phone. To my surprise, they did, and I rattled off my presentation to the doctor, hopeful they would continue the work up with compassion.

"Her rash is consistent with leukemia, and she needs a stat blood count with a manual differential and peripheral blood smear; I hate to send them through the ER if you can order that outpatient in the morning for—"

I was cut off by her crisp voice and a dial tone in quick succession, "Yeah, just send them to the ER."

So much for the kindly pediatrician.

I went back to the room and steadied myself with a kinder version of the truth, "Alright, mamma, pediatrician agrees with me that she should be seen in an emergency setting because of the rash and fatigue. I'll write up a summary as to why I'm sending you, give you a copy of the packet, and call them in advance so they have your ETA."

To my surprise, she was not upset, she was invigorated, "Thank you! Thank you for listening. I knew something wasn't right."

"Listen, I don't know what's going to happen tonight, but please know that you did a good job following your instincts by getting a second opinion. Whatever this is, it isn't normal and you're going to go to the right place to figure out what comes next."

She hugged me and as I watched them leave my clinic, I sent a silent secular prayer into the night with them. I hoped the child would be alright. I hoped at least one of us would be alright.

The next morning, the mother called to let me know her daughter was admitted to the inpatient pediatric ward for Acute Lymphoblastic Leukemia.

She was starting chemotherapy that week.

Because You're Nice to Me

To dismiss is simple, but to care is complex.

My personal philosophy of medicine is that it is my role to provide my patients with the education and resources to make the best-informed decisions for themselves. It is not my role to judge, but rather to facilitate. The importance of kindness underscores true healing, as all too often clinicians dismiss what they do not understand and they do so unkindly. Clinical arrogance hides ignorance but I believe there is no place for the ego at the bedside.

As my health continued to deteriorate, I focused on the care of my patients. I threw myself into clinical cases in the hope that someone would get something good out of their interactions with me. I didn't care about my personal relationships and, as far as I was concerned, the worse the pain got, the less I cared about myself.

"He's back," the manager scoffed as somebody diagnosed with Munchausen's was checked in at registration.

I cast an angry look their way but remained silent. I knew there wasn't much I could say to dissuade her from speaking ill of anyone she chose, and she was a bit vindictive, so it was best to stay off her radar. I wasn't looking to get into fights with coworkers and certainly wanted to avoid middle management's ire. The patient in question was a challenging one, but one of my favorites. He was only nineteen years old and heavily medicated on antipsychotics. The medications caused his belly and face to balloon up with more than just baby fat, and he was prone to fits of rage.

The first time I met him, his grandfather dropped him off at the clinic and sped away. It was only later I found out this was a regular pattern. The patriarch hoped that, by abandoning him, we would transfer the patient to yet another psych facility or inpatient holding cell.

"What's he here for this time?" I asked the medical assistant.

"Sliced arms. Not too deep. You can get away with bandaging them, but it'll take forever cuz he did both of 'em again." The medical assistant shrugged. "I laid out what ya need but kept the sharps locked because of last time."

Last time he tried to steal a few scalpels and a few needles because he was prone to inserting them into his blossoming belly fat. Once, I was told, he inserted a 22-gauge needle but it broke off at the base, and he lost it in the fold. The urgent care provider on shift yelled at him for coming to their location and told him he was outright crazy. He grinned with tears in his eyes as the ambulance took him away, according to the support staff.

After I introduced myself, I sat down and looked appraisingly at his pale, flabby arms. He was a bloody Zebra, and my heart broke for him.

"Does it hurt?"

"Not really." He tilted his head to the side, judging me. "Felt good. You know?"

I knew. I had been picking at my skin for years, as long as I could remember. I didn't consider it self-mutilation then; I simply considered it a family habit I picked up from dear old dad. Dad was constantly ripping at his skin, blooms of red blossoming on his arms and legs, anywhere his fingers could reach to release the nervousness.

"Not much to suture up here; you didn't go too deep."

"I know."

As I pulled out the supplies to bandage him, I asked, "What happened to trigger it?"

He lit up and his story came out in pressured tones. Instead of shushing him or rushing through the wound care, I took my time, and I listened. I was curious and he was the most interesting case I had seen all day. Besides, at that time I was lucky enough to have an empty lobby, so there was no reason to rush him at all. The first time he told me he had Munchausen's, he laughed when I expressed disbelief that he identified it so willingly to me.

"Aren't you supposed to trick me into caring for you?" I smiled wryly at the sardonic teen on my table.

"You're caring for me right now, aren't you?" He smiled back, waving the already wrapped left arm.

Technically, Munchausen's is a colloquial term, and the proper diagnosis is Factitious Disorder Imposed on Self. This refers to a pervasive pattern of deceptively misrepresenting, simulating, or causing symptoms of an illness even in the absence of obvious external rewards (such as financial gain, housing, or medications). Factitious Disorder by proxy, formerly known as Munchausen's by proxy, refers to intentionally hurting another while you take them for medical care. In this young man's case, no one was hurting him intentionally; he was the one doing it.

He admitted he knew exactly why he was prone to exaggerate these symptoms. When this teenager was a toddler, he experienced the opposite of medical trauma. He experienced what it was like for someone to be kind to him in a medical setting. When he was only six years old, he had a cyst on his kidney that required surgery. His home life was abusive, so when he was a kid in recovery, propped up with clean, heated blankets and given popsicles whenever he hit a button, he was hooked.

He wanted to be a patient forever, and he eventually got his wish.

He hated going home to a mother that hit him and a father that drank too much, so he started injuring himself in various ways to get the attention of the pediatrician. Unfortunately, his parents and grandfather realized this would only lead to legal woes for them, so they often ignored his pain until it was life or limb threatening. This resulted in increasingly escalating behavior that wound him up in various urgent cares and emergency rooms, but rarely the same ones to avoid a paper trail.

He started cutting himself around the age of nine.

He started burning himself around the age of eleven.

He started experiencing seizures around the age of fourteen.

By the time he was properly diagnosed with an underlying etiology, Frontal Lobe Epilepsy, he had already been medicated with more sedatives than a psych ward and had more recovery surgeries than anyone I've yet to meet in my lifetime. He had real pain, and he was leaning into it in the most unhealthy ways.

He kept coming back to me and I kept treating him nicely.

Even when the staff scoffed, I remained steadfast in my care for him. One day, I said to him only half-jokingly, "You know, we need to stop meeting like this."

He giggled.

"When are you going to stop hurting yourself?" At this point in our relationship, I could be blunt. He knew about my growing abdominal pain and would give me a chance to rest during our visits. The first time he saw my breath catch, he called me out, curious because he recognized the hints of pain just below the socially acceptable surface. He asked if I was OK and I told him that I wasn't but we were there for him, not the other way around.

Spending extra time on a complex wound care psych patient is a great way to steal a five-to-ten-minute break for yourself in the urgent care. He didn't judge me when I needed to take a few deep breaths to steady my hand before continuing with his ministrations. He held space for me in the same way I held space for him and, in a strange way, we were umbrellas for each other offering a temporary break from the expectations outside the clinic room.

"I dunno; maybe if this new doctor can save me."

He had an appointment coming up in the next month with a new neurologist. He was hopeful he was going to take his fits of rage and self-harm of evidence that his Frontal Lobe Epilepsy was not well controlled and that he did, in fact, need real medical help.

Not just because he was bored and lonely.

I warned him against looking for a savior in medicine; I had decades and degrees on him, and I was still waiting for mine. We were both waiting for a physician priest who would absolve us of our genetic sins but I was slowly losing my faith.

At that point, the weight was steadily falling off at a rate of two to three pounds a week. Food was becoming a significant issue for me, and I found myself resentful of my husband's delightful cooking because I could no longer participate. He tried, god how he tried, by changing up our standard meals into soups and stews with the hopes that I'd absorb some of that goodness.

I found the process of consuming anything increasingly painful. To avoid running to the bathroom mid-shift, I started intentionally starving myself. If I didn't eat, the pain was replaced by searing, hollow hunger instead of debilitating regurgitation.

Another one of my patients, Magpie, a seventy-something-year-old sweetheart, kept coming by long after I repaired her skin tears. She was a skinny thing, but her head was crowned with a frizzled mop of brown ringlets and her personality was larger than life. She considered herself a grandmother to the community, and, once she met me and my crew, she decided to take us under her wing. Like my Munchausen's patient, she too understood pain and could tell something was brewing in my belly that wasn't good so she'd bring us treats.

Every few weeks, she would swing by with bags of chips or chocolates under her scrawny arms, eager to sit for a spell and share stories about the Vermont of her youth. When she first moved to the rural area between Burlington and Canada, her family was scorned.

"Vermont's always been a racist place," she explained between bites of lobster roll potato chips. "Ha! They called me a half-breed!"

She went on to explain that she was a proud Italian, but, because of her family's darker skin, the locals assumed they were black. The experience provided her with a profound sense of understanding of what it meant to be discriminated against and so, as she aged, she used her ability to pass between worlds to build bridges between them. She volunteered her time to the sick and the infirm, and that continued well into when I knew her.

One day, she stopped by and complimented my weight loss. "You're looking good! Feeling good?"

"No, not really," I replied.

She frowned, her crab-apple face wrinkling further. "I worry about you. I'm going to start bringing you more food, and you better eat it! You work too hard!"

It was when I was chomping on some of her lobster roll potato chips that the cousin of the leukemia girl got checked in with his grandfather in tow. As I've said, you get to know families when you work in rural medicine, and this place was no different. I'd built a practice in this place even though my corporate overlords couldn't care less about anything other than the bottom line.

The thirteen-year-old boy was husky and hunched over, his double chin dripping with saliva. He was endorsing 10/10 abdominal pain, which started the night prior, just after family dinner, without fevers, vomiting, or diarrhea. The grandfather was at a loss because everyone else in the family had the same simple meal, fried chicken and baked beans, but Cousin here was just all out of sorts.

His vital signs showed an elevated heart rate and slightly elevated blood pressure, which wasn't unexpected as he was an obese kiddo and was clearly in pain. His soft, white belly groaned with hyperactive bowel sounds, and I asked him when his last bowel movement was. He confirmed the day before.

"And the last thing you ate?"

His grandfather quipped, "You already asked that; I told ya."

"Yes, but he didn't." I pointed at the boy, guilt blossoming across his face as he turned to look away.

"Boy?" the grandfather asked sternly. "You got something you hiding? You get into the cakes again?"

"No!" he yelped a little too quickly.

Like most teenagers, he had secrets, and one of his secrets was his love of McDonald's. One of his older buddies, who had a car and less aware parents, dropped off a secret order after the rest of his family went to bed. After he ate the family meal of fried chicken and baked beans, this boy had:

Two double bacon cheeseburgers

Three orders of large fries

Twenty chicken nuggets

Two large colas

Two apple pies

By the time we finished calculating the kid's intake, we realized he had binged something like 10,000 calories, resulting in the worst tummy ache of his life. We gave him a GI cocktail in the clinic, which was a mixture of viscous lidocaine, Maalox, and Benadryl, and we waited.

And waited.

And then he erupted.

His grandfather and I sat in the exam room, listening to the soft moans of relief wash over the kid in the bathroom, and I suggested they keep a closer eye on his nighttime activities. The grandfather admitted he was acting out more since his cousin was diagnosed with leukemia, and we spent some time talking about how tough it can be for the healthy ones.

Survivor's guilt is real and sometimes we strike out to find control in the unhealthiest of ways.

I thought of my family watching me waste away, and how unreachable I had been despite everyone's kindness. Just like that little boy emptying his bowels and the teenager hoping for a neurological savior, I was just suffering while waiting for salvation. I was also becoming increasingly blind to those who were around me offering help.

Magpie was right to be worried, but no amount of potato chips could hold off what was coming next.

Is That Blood?

"Is that blood?"

My blue emesis bag swirled with chunks of what looked like coffee grounds after a particularly painful retching episode. I wiped my mouth and struggled to catch my breath though it was difficult to take in anything beyond shallow gulps of air. After a few moments, my head pounding and my heart racing, I opened the bathroom door, looking for my husband.

He saw me holding the heavy blue bag and I asked him weakly, "Does this look like blood to you?"

He shook his head in the negative, reassuring me it was likely just chocolate. I was eating a ton of chocolate at that point. With my stomach persistently and consistently rejecting food after food, I found myself gravitating toward things that would melt in my mouth: chocolate Boost shakes, chocolate squares, whole milk lattes, crackers, and ice cream. Certainly not a healthy diet by any stretch of the imagination, but it was the only thing getting me through.

I was a clinician running on caffeine, chocolate, and cannabis...and a lot of desperation. Those student loans continued to choke me month after month, and we found ourselves maxing out every credit card we owned on medical bills. As the main breadwinner of the family, I couldn't skip out on shifts because as an urgent care provider I was a contract worker paid hourly with bare bones benefits. I justified dragging myself out of bed every day despite the pain by telling myself that if I could continue to rack in the hours at a white-collar hourly rate, what did it matter how much pain I was in?

For me, my life didn't matter very much at all.

I insisted, shoving the bag toward him, "What about coffee grounds? Does it look like ground coffee?"

Again, he reassured me it was likely just the dark-colored foods I'd attempted to eat earlier in the day. I didn't have the energy to debate so I dismissed my symptom with the logic my husband presented in front of me. It did fit. I didn't have a successful shift from a calorie or hydration standpoint, but my corporate overlords placed me in one of the less busy clinics and therefore we were chronically short staffed. I was lucky to have a receptionist and a medical assistant, and often was tasked with working just one-to-one which meant no one got breaks.

That night, I chose to go to sleep early in an attempt to get rest for my next shift, less than twelve hours away. I put myself to bed, an emesis bag within reach, and left my husband to the green glow of digital guns and video games.

A few hours later, I jolted upright, choking on thick, hot blood, sputtering in the dark. I emptied my guts into the blue bag at my bedside, eyes bulging and stomach screaming in agony. The retching finally stopped, and I stumbled out of bed, hit the lights, and saw the streaks of red swirling in the depths of the plastic and all over my bed.

Mallory Weiss tears are most common in alcoholics and occur after a particularly violent retching episode.

A little piece of medical trivia wafted to the forefront of my mind, but I couldn't remember what came after because I was hit with another wave of retching, flecks of red dotting my hands further.

Motherfucker: That is blood.

I knew exactly what was wrong with me: I suffered a Mallory Weiss tear. While it is true these are most commonly seen in alcoholics, any injury in which the intrathoracic and abdominal pressures are acutely raised can trigger a vessel rupture. And that's all it was: a burst vessel in my esophagus.

Just like when we cough forcefully and pop a blood vessel in our eye (temporarily turning into the Living Dead with a blood-shot visage), we can pop other vessels. It's when you pop the big ones, like the ones lining your already inflamed esophagus, that you run into problems. In my case, my stomach was filling up with the steady ooze of venous blood and I couldn't empty it because of the gastroparesis. Therefore, the blood was curdling in my belly and then forcefully erupting back up out of my mouth and into the world.

This was a different agony than my daily dose of pain from gastroparesis. That left me feeling hollow and empty. This pain was something entirely different, a new breed of dragon that had come from the depths of my gene pool to haunt me. I didn't know how to fight this one off, so I didn't hesitate to go to the Emergency Room and check myself with a chief complaint of "Vomiting Blood."

We waited.

Then we waited some more.

Sitting in an emergency room triage as a clinician in pain is an interesting experience indeed. I used the patients around me as case studies in distraction. The woman across from me was curled up on a dilapidated wheelchair, half her body folding into the other half while her adult daughter desperately jabbered into the phone, lamenting her mother was still in the lobby even after her imaging study. It was clear to me the woman had suffered a stroke at some point in her journey and it was likely her current state wasn't a significant change above her baseline, but try explaining that bit of medical callousness to the average Jane.

She ain't having it.

Next to me, a man had a blood clot in his left lower leg. He had been waiting for three hours, even though his Primary Care Doctor had told him to go earlier in the day. As I eavesdropped on his conversation with his emaciated wife, I learned he had complained of swelling in his calf to his PCP that morning, but, in his eagerness to dismiss the diagnosis, the patient decided to wait it out at home and see if "it got better on its own." When the swelling worsened and he developed frank pain in his calf, he started to worry. He couldn't sleep, so he and the Missus ended up next to us in that fateful lobby that night. He just couldn't understand why he had to wait so long.

As I curled up in my own ball, losing all sense of dignity and collapsing to the floor while my husband listened for my name, I realized all of us would be waiting for a very long time.

Finally, at the peak of my exhaustion, I was brought back to a bay, and my intake began.

None of the clinical staff knew what gastroparesis was, and I struggled to repeat the same script to each new staff member. No one spoke to one another either, and no one really understood what was said anyway. It was infuriating.

The nurse side-eyed me as I mentioned I used medical marijuana for the pain, and I felt stabs of shame while my stomach continued its assault. I was labeled a drug seeker before the physician even laid eyes on me, and I knew this would be an upward battle. She made some offhand comment about causing the nausea myself by smoking too much weed but I didn't have the energy to educate her.

When the resident came in, I weakly presented my case to him, "I have a Mallory-Weiss tear…"

"We'll see about that." He interrupted me with what seemed like a pathetic attempt to reassure me, "It's our job to diagnose you and oftentimes what patients think is vomiting blood is really just nothing at all."

I took a jagged breath. I steeled myself for this fool, reminding myself he didn't know what he didn't know, but goddamn was it invalidating. I didn't have the energy to hold my head up, never mind argue with his dismissal before he so much as palpated my abdomen or took my pulse.

This resident represented all that was wrong with medical education at that moment in time: ego, ego, ego.

I tried again, giving him a detailed history of present illness, so much so that all the poor man had to do was go outside my room, regurgitate it to his attending, and wait for her to finish the assessment. When his attending did attend to me, I found her bedside manner to be pleasant, and she offered me a modicum of respect when she realized I practiced up the street in the outpatient urgent care.

She still didn't listen to me, though.

She pushed morphine when I specifically told her not to do so.

It's ironic, almost. So many of my fellow gastroparesis warriors would go into emergency rooms all over the world, begging for help for various complications, and they'd be accused of drug-seeking and malingering. They'd be turned away with Tylenol and a tsk-tsking of the staff. So many of the friends I've met on my medical journey would never be offered pain management even at their most painful apexes, and here I was telling this doctor I didn't want the morphine.

So, what did I want?

I wanted it to stop.

I was beyond logic, but I knew I wanted the pain to stop, however that may be possible.

I suggested Tylenol and Toradol, knowing we could use a combination of injectable and rectal medications to bypass my fickle stomach. The attending reassured me I'd be fine, but as I watched the morphine descend into my vein, I braced myself for the drug reaction. If you've never had a morphine push before, the best way I can describe it for me is that it felt like a burning flush that rose in the back of my throat and traveled through my veins and spine. It felt like fire and the nausea crested in a new wave.

I retched fruitfully.

A bounty of blood spilled forth into the kidney dish held on my lap, and in an almost triumphant manner, I turned to the medical team as if to say, "*See? I wasn't lying. I'm not a drug seeker. I'm not a monster. I'm a woman in pain goddammit.*"

Of course, I didn't say any of those things out loud. I was still too afraid to speak up too much. I was afraid of being labeled an aggressive patient or even worse, a hypochondriac. Especially considering I worked with these people by proxy. When I had a case that was too complex for my city urgent care post, I'd turf them upward and onward to their Emergency Room. They knew my name outside of my patient chart, and I had my name on file with their HR as a potential hire for future spots.

I wanted to be perceived as a compliant patient.

As I vomited again in front of the team, the attending nodded, realizing my diagnosis was likely correct. When she said she would admit me to the hospital for observation, I panicked. I realized I hadn't coordinated coverage for the shift the next morning. That morning. I was expected to be at work in six hours. It was understood that if a provider didn't find coverage for their clinic, the entire site would be shut down for the day and none of the staff paid.

I can't describe the conflict this presented accurately. My staff were dependent on their paychecks. A single shift missed could make or break a family's monthly budget, and with each mounting medical bill, I was feeling the same crunch.

"What will you do for me if I'm admitted?"

The attending was taken aback, but, before she could question my judgment, I explained, "If I don't show up to work tomorrow, no one gets paid. My staff won't get paid."

She stated I'd be signing out against her recommendations. She wanted to put me on nothing by mouth, also known as NPO, so my esophagus could heal. They would monitor my vital signs, likely replace more fluids, and I would get a gastroenterology consult in the morning. And if need be, the site would be cauterized.

I told her that I wouldn't eat anything by mouth and I'd call my gastroenterologist when his office opened. I told her I needed to report to work and at least if I crashed while on shift, theoretically my urgent care staff could call an ambulance to bring me right back up the street to her Emergency Room. My vitals were stable, and I was an adult with sound medical reasoning backed by a license. She couldn't hold me, nor would she want to; beds were always short and quick turnover is praised. Besides, from a liability standpoint, the emergency room physician was cleared because she could document my history and reasoning behind the discharge over admission.

"Are you sure you're going to be OK?" she asked, genuinely as one woman to another, as my husband left me alone to get the car.

165

"My staff will help me out. I'll try to keep it as a light day." I avoided answering her question directly.

I should have listened to her and stayed. I should have been stabilized. I should have submitted to an inpatient gastroenterology consult, because maybe then I would have gotten the imaging I needed. But, I didn't, and I pushed myself to the very brink because of money.

We were short staffed that day.

It was not a light day at all.

As I kept myself from eating or drinking a single sip of anything, I took care of thirty-seven outpatient urgent care patients, all praying for someone to listen as I used them to distract me from my pain.

Kidney Stoned to Death

Perhaps if I went to sleep one day, I might get lucky and never wake up.

The intrusive thoughts were getting darker by the day.

My husband and I were fighting more than usual, naturally, as he had become no longer a partner or a lover, but a caregiver, and our relationship suffered. We both knew what it was like to live with chronic pain, but, as my condition continued to deteriorate, neither of us understood how I could become so pathetic. When I got off a shift, I had so little energy left I could barely wash my hair. I had to rely on him for everything and once I fell onto the couch or bed, I wasn't getting back up again until it was time to work, because of the pain.

But, when we think of pain, clinicians tend to rank it on a scale of zero to ten. It's a horrifically faulty scale because numbers can never explain what it feels like to die. To survive dying.

When I'd walk into an exam room with a patient eating Hot Cheetos endorsing 10/10 belly pain, I knew the scale was faulty. When I experienced my first kidney stone, I knew the scale was faulty. I couldn't verbalize when I was at 10/10. I couldn't sustain consciousness when I was at 10/10. I certainly couldn't explain anything.

When you reach a certain threshold of pain, it's easier to submit. It's easier to fall into unconsciousness, and that's exactly what happened to me the night I was kidney stoned to death. My husband and I were eagerly planning a trip to Maine, filled with duck fat fries (as I was still able to eat French fries!) followed by sea kayaking for him. I didn't have the energy to splash around on the open water. Instead, I was planning on enjoying a reflexology session at a tea-themed salon with a good book while he conquered the salted waves.

I worked the previous five shifts in a row and it was obvious that I was dehydrated but I put a paper-thin smile on and told myself I was fine. I just needed a good night's sleep before our vacation. I woke in the early morning hours with a dull ache in my right flank and told my husband I thought I was getting my period. I went to the bathroom to sit on the toilet and pray it would pass. I didn't want to miss out on those fries.

I sat next to the white porcelain throne, alternating sitting on the toilet with diarrhea and laying my head against the soaking tub with only a towel between myself and the cold tile. I licked my dry lips, daydreaming about salt and fat and I felt wave after wave of pain bubble up from my lower belly and back until I faded to black.

"Wake up! Holy shit, wake up!" My husband found me sprawled out on the floor, a few hours later, cold to the touch and mumbling gibberish.

I opened my eyes and realized I had passed out at some point, but time was like taffy; it was stretching in an alien way I'd never experienced before in my life. I felt cold. I asked him to help me back onto the toilet from the floor. I remember his eyes wrinkled in concern. I remember him locking our Labrador retriever into his crate so the paramedics could get into our apartment without him underfoot. I remember laughing ironically as he cried, I was grateful it was an all-female team that greeted me half naked and more than half dead. I was delirious.

As they bounced me into the ambulance, I whispered, "I swear I'm not a drug seeker, but can I get something for the pain?"

The paramedic ignored (or didn't hear) me, instead yelling to the driver, "I can't get peripheral access; not getting a BP either!"

"In that case," I joked using my last breath, "I'm going to go to sleep now."

My eyes fluttered, offering glimpses of upside-down traffic lights followed quickly by upside down hospital lights, the fluorescent bulbs searing my eyes and reinforcing my desire to stay asleep. I didn't want to wake up. I wanted to stay in the in between waking and passing; I didn't care if that meant passing out or passing away. I wanted to stay blissfully unaware of the men and women poking my body with needles and spreading my legs.

A nurse repeatedly smacked my left arm and in response, it trembled.

Jacksonian March?

My train of thought stopped as soon as it started, and the nurse asked me if I'd ever experienced that kind of localized seizure activity before. "When I was a kid…"

Before I could respond to her further, I felt my legs being re-positioned bluntly as a pelvic wedge was placed below. Two men, one of whom looked vaguely familiar, popped up between my legs and I felt the familiar intrusion of cold plastic and lubricating jelly.

"Ughhh." I groaned but couldn't fully verbalize as the men withdrew their instruments and fingers.

"Let's send her for pelvic ultrasound…"

I didn't hear the rest. My husband filled in the blanks for me, later. I took several IV bags of fluid to return to consciousness, and my electrolytes were all out of whack. Misbehaving magnesium and problematic potassium would become a trend for me as I continued to bounce in and out of emergency rooms.

My husband was told, "Call the family."

When a provider tells a patient's family member to call the rest of the family, that usually only means one thing: it's time to say goodbye. Reading through my discharge paperwork days later though, you'd never know I was at death's door. Despite my husband telling me the paramedics recorded a core body temperature of 93 degrees, despite my recollection of passing out and the excruciating pain that preceded it, the ER paperwork simply listed my diagnosis as:

Abdominal Pain NOS (Not Otherwise Specified)

Nowhere was there documentation of my gastroparesis, or the strange case of ketones in my urine without any sign of diabetes. When I finally regained coherent consciousness, the ER doctor literally scratched his head as he explained to me that he didn't know what was wrong with me, but he could tell something was really wrong with me. He couldn't explain my collapse. He said he just couldn't put his finger on it. In the meantime, he could refill my Zofran for nausea and advised me I should think about seeing a specialist.

My husband and I spent somewhere around twelve hours dealing with the kidney stone from hell. The only reason I can point to a more concrete diagnosis than Abdominal Pain NOS (which I consider a lazy placeholder), is because I reviewed my CT scan and surmised that the presence of kidney stones in both kidneys meant it was likely I had an obstruction earlier in the night which caused me to go into a renal colic episode.

In a healthy patient, kidney stones and renal colic are considered some of the most painful conditions one can experience. The most painful medical condition is generally agreed to be end-stage pancreatic cancer, but that's a different story. Treatment for these poor writhing kidney stone souls includes forcing tons of fluids to flush the kidneys, pain control with good old-fashioned Tylenol and Motrin, and in some cases prescription medications to relax the ureter.

While I was able to walk out of the hospital that day, we still didn't have an answer for why I couldn't compensate for any acute illnesses or injuries. A kidney stone nearly killed me and, while that doctor didn't realize why I had ketones in my urine, I did:

I was starving to death.

Did You Ski Last Year?

When you're starving to death, the world feels translucent.

Like the paper we use to line exam tables; it's there but it will rip with just the slightest shift.

I was more zombie than woman at this point, punching in and out, but completely clocked out.

I was contemplating when I'd finally say it was enough but I didn't tell anyone that's where my thoughts were going. I was entertaining some suicidal fantasies at this point, but they were fleeting. They were sparks behind closed eyelids when the vomiting got me close to syncope. They were intrusive thoughts that came out when I wasn't distracted by my medical practice. They were whispers in the dark when I didn't want to shit myself in bed. They were prayers, of a kind, hoping for release.

If I was a zombie, I was a zombie praying for a grave to finally claim me.

Work continued to grind heavy on my bony shoulders, as I was working alone and in an isolated setting. I had no colleagues to compare notes with, unless I reached out to distant sites an hour plus away via telephone, and, in my isolation, I grew more and more convinced I was a terrible clinician. I couldn't save my-self and therefore I believed I couldn't save anyone else.

The most common intrusive thought told me: *I was a piece of shit.*

Our corporate overlords continued to demand more out of us with increasingly fewer resources and staffing in urgent care. I can't count the shifts I staffed with only one or two employees with me. We were expected to juggle any case that came through the doors and have the patients happily served and out in under an hour. Medicine is rarely what people want, so to add on time constraints and customer satisfaction scores when the overall goal of urgent care is to triage and direct just didn't compute. Patients were frustrated. I was frustrated.

You're a piece of shit, a voice hissed out of the growing dark-ness. *You're a fucking piece of shit fraud.*

This wasn't a new voice, but it was a voice that only came out in my darkest moments. It spat out various scripts of sadness tinged with pure poison. It was Imposter Syndrome incarnate, the worst part of my internal dialogue made masculine, and it was manifesting itself more and more often.

You're a fraud.

You have no idea what you're doing.

You couldn't save yourself as a kid, how could you save yourself now?

These thoughts were heavy on my mind as the electronic med-ical record lit up with a new patient. A seventy-six-year-old woman, Jean, checked in for "heartburn," but any clinician worth their salt knows that women present with cardiac issues in a variety of ways. Indigestion, fatigue, unexplained nausea, and chest pressure are all red flags.

I entered the room quickly and conducted a cardiopulmonary exam. She held her fist above her chest, raising it up and down, completing a classic Levine's Sign as she said, "It's just like an elephant is sitting on my chest but the Tums aren't helping."

My assistant was already prepping the EKG machine outside the exam room, and I advised her that I'd like to get an EKG reading, administer some aspirin, and call 911 for transport to a local hospital with a cardiac center. Granted that local hospital was still a good thirty minutes away, and, if my suspicions were right and she was having a cardiac event, time was tissue.

She scoffed. "It's just indigestion!"

"That's what my mom said during her first heart attack and I don't think this is a case where you want to be wrong," I countered.

She patted my arm in a measured, kind way and reassured me. "I can't be having a heart attack. I went skiing last year and I'm getting ready to go again this fall."

"Be that as it may—"

"Did *you* ski last year?" She interrupted, pointedly crossing her arms with more of a playful smirk than anything else.

I admitted I didn't because of my own health issues and, after a few minutes of bargaining, she consented to the EKG to "prove me wrong."

She was having a heart attack.

The squiggly lines were raised in all the wrong places, suggesting she was experiencing a STEMI, also known as an ST- segment elevated myocardial infarction.

As the lead paramedic reviewed the rhythm strip he whispered to me, "Holy shit, this might be *the* big one for her."

"I know," I whispered back. "Get her out of here and where she needs to be."

I didn't want her dying in my clinic. She trusted me enough to run the test that confirmed my diagnosis, and she trusted me enough to go onward to the next step of treatment. Even though the vicious whispers were starting to become stronger, meeting Jean felt like a sign. Sometimes, you are in the right place at the right time, and an intervention saves you. Even though the path is crooked, there can be redemption if only you have enough faith to trust there are still people out there willing to help.

She waved weakly as the men rolled her out of my clinic and into the cool air outside.

I wondered if I'd ever see her again.

I also wondered, strangely, if I'd ever be healthy enough to ski again. But before I could stop the vicious voice from bubbling up again, it hissed from the depths:

You're never going to be healthy again.

From Gunner to Gun Shy

"He said he was going to shoot us all," my medical receptionist blurted with eyes wide.

I looked back at the elderly man in exam room one complaining of food poisoning and his adult son and smiled briskly, hoping they didn't hear what was just said in the hallway. I closed the exam door and put my back against it bracing myself as I took stock of the outpatient urgent care clinic.

It was thirty minutes to close and our retail facility was staffed with four women, myself included. The parking lot was dark and the streetlamp flickered casting shadows as I looked out the front doors. I realized with a sinking feeling the entire clinic was surrounded by glass. The only entrance to the clinic was a recessed glass front door after an external glass door. Once inside the lobby, an assailant could easily jump over the receptionist's desk or walk through the double doors into the clinic because none of our internal doors locked. We were sitting ducks.

"Call 911." I inhaled sharply.

I had two families in the clinic; thankfully we weren't at capacity. First, I knocked on the door of the patient I had not seen yet; it was a mother with two young children. I quickly informed them of the situation and advised them to shelter in place. She looked at me as though I was absolutely nuts, grabbed her kids, and sprinted out into the parking lot, driving away before anything could happen.

I wished I could drive away, too.

I went back to my food poisoning patient. He couldn't flee. He was hooked up to an IV receiving fluids.

I cautioned the patient and his adult son, "No matter what you hear outside, I need you to stay in this room as quietly as possible. We have just received a credible active shooter threat. Police are on their way."

The elderly man with the IV didn't say a word but his son simply let an "Oh" leak out. It was like a deflating balloon.

As I closed the door, I felt myself leaving my body in shock as I sheltered in place in the back office, wondering which armed man would show up first, police or perpetrator.

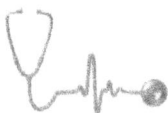

Saying no to men is tricky.

It's much easier to say yes, and then convince them they didn't want the thing after all.

In medicine, though, sometimes you have to say no to people. In fact, I say it a lot. Whether it is someone requesting an inappropriate prescription, often narcotic in nature, or it is a mother asking for an inappropriate exception, often vaccine in nature, clinicians must remain strong. We can't be swayed by emotional manipulations or threats or bribes. We must focus on the evidence, present the information to the patient, and coordinate the care they both want and need.

It can never be just what they want.

And it should never be just what they need.

Months earlier, at a different urgent care in a more rural setting, I received a credible threat of violence from a different man. I couldn't believe this was happening to me again. The first time, the patient was a white man approaching eighty years old, and his breath stank of burnt tobacco and fermenting apples. He walked with a slight impairment in his left leg, and he squinted when he spoke, crust gathering at his eyes. You didn't need a white coat to recognize he was not a healthy man.

So, it raised serious questions when I looked over his Commercial Driver's License exam form and found his medical history was a series of stone cold "NOs." How could a man in his eighth decade of life be unscathed by the progress of time and the inevitable addition of pharmaceutical interventions?

The answer was he wasn't, and he was committing medical fraud.

He lied up and down about his health history.

Unfortunately, this was only the first red flag, as he also refused to enter the exam room alone, insisting his wife accompany him. There's no reason for your spouse to join you on a federally mandated physical exam, and I find that individuals who bring visitors are often looking to distract the clinician. He forgot his glasses, so my medical assistant informed him that we recommended he pause his examination to go get his glasses (at home,

178

according to him). In the meantime, we asked who his primary care provider was so we could fax his card over to them when we were done.

He provided her contact information and, cussing us up and down, he left to go "get his goddamn glasses."

When you certify a commercial driver, you need to be willing to put your license on the line that this person is safe to drive several tons of metal at speeds approaching eighty miles an hour. You need to be willing to bet not your life, but theirs, and the lives of those on the road around them.

Out of everything I can do for a patient in the world of medicine, commercial driver licenses examinations are among my least favorite appointments.

I would go so far as to say I hate them.

I hate them more than I hated Christmas as a kid.

It's because sometimes I have to tell a person that they have diabetes, or uncontrollable blood pressure and they are not qualified to drive a commercial vehicle. This wouldn't be such a big issue if the patient wasn't then at risk of losing their health insurance because in America, our employers often dictate our access to medical care. When these people leave my office without a driver's license card in hand, they are sometimes losing their ability to generate income.

Sometimes this means they lose their job and sometimes this means they lose their house because many people are living paycheck to paycheck in America.

So, no, I did not trust this aggressive elderly man and his wife with the pinched face because he had valid motivation to lie on his form. I did not trust his eyesight was the only thing amiss about his health, and I took the opportunity to call his primary care physician while he was out of my office on that glasses task.

To my great surprise, the receptionist snorted when I said the patient's name and patched me right through to the doctor. No waiting. Red flag number two wasn't just raised, it was on fire. It was rare to be patched through that quickly in the middle of a clinic day, so that told me that this patient was well known by his primary care office. Once she got on the line, not only did she inform me that she refused to even entertain a commercial driver's license appointment with him, but she also couldn't write a letter for me to clear him.

He was not medically certifiable.

He was also actively being investigated for a DUI. The doctor warned me he was fired from their practice because he was a raging alcoholic with an aggressive streak and a collection of guns at home. She wished me good luck before hanging up. I blinked looking at the receiver and prayed he wouldn't return.

Of course, he returned.

I told my manager I was concerned he had the potential to turn aggressive and, thankfully, Tony listened. He was a good man and a former army medic, so I felt safe with him standing just outside the door, but we were all on full alert. We kept the exam room door slightly ajar. We had the receptionist ready to call 911 if things got difficult. We were ready for his aggression, and that made all the difference in this particular case.

When he returned, I greeted him up front, took him back immediately, and advised the patient that we didn't need to do an eye examination. I continued and gently explained that I had spoken to his primary care provider after he left, and she had updated me on his health status. I didn't even have a chance to explain that, as a federally mandated exam it was out of my hands, before he stood up screaming.

"That BITCH," he snarled. "She's a liar!"

I stood up and backed away, never taking my eyes off him, and Tony opened the exam room door fully so the patient understood I was not without backup.

"I'm so sorry, I know this is hard—"

"You don't know shit. You're killing me." He took a few steps toward the door, but lingered, wringing his hands. "You don't know what you're doing to me."

"I'm sorry. I can't certify you based on—"

"We'll lose everything."

"I know but—"

"You don't know anything! She's a liar, I'm fine. I drove here, didn't I?" He continued ranting, desperately looking for a way to walk out of the clinic with the card that could keep him punching in and out of his day job.

There's a certain kind of heartbreak that festers when you condemn a man to poverty. It's worse when he could be your grandfather.

Until he threatens to kill you.

"You're taking my life. I'm coming back for you with my shotgun and I'm going to take your life. I'm going to take everything away from you like you're doing to me." His eyes bored into mine as he cursed me.

"That's enough." Tony stepped in, and escorted the man out.

I didn't want to be a statistic, and yet there I was, standing in the middle of a rural clinic waiting for a disgruntled patient to come back to "take my life."

Tony took all appropriate steps to ensure our safety that day. Initially, upper management advised us to make a note of it in his medical chart and move on. I was told to shake it off. That it probably was hot air and that I was being dramatic if I really thought the patient would return. I should just get over it and I really didn't need to escalate it to involve the police. Tony disagreed with the corporation's response and supported me in filing a police report that very day.

The judge granted me a restraining order within a week. At the end of the day, a restraining order is just a piece of paper and can't protect anyone from a bullet. But it felt like something. And in medicine, I've learned the power of suggestion is magical. When you give patients something to do to fix their problem, they feel like they have some semblance of control.

Even if it's all smoke and mirrors.

Especially when it's all smoke and mirrors.

The old man in the rural clinic never came back so I suppose the restraining order was effective. Now, months later I was facing another disgruntled man, this time younger and significantly more motivated than the old man before him. I darkly wondered if my company would accuse us of all being dramatic this time as well.

We cowered at our desks and watched the dark parking lot with various mixed emotions. One of my unhinged medical assistants started to sympathize with the would-be-shooter. She started agreeing with his philosophy, saying we did charge patients too much and we deserved whatever we got. I wanted to tell her to shut up but someone else did before I could.

We asked the receptionist over and over again what the young man on the telephone said exactly. He was mad that he needed to pay for an appointment this evening. He was very mad that I wouldn't call an antibiotic in for him even though the receptionist explained that I had never met him before and we do not prescribe medication over the phone. He apparently told her that he would come to the clinic, not with money, but with his guns loaded to give us "what we deserve".

The receptionist was shaken up because she said she could also hear a woman arguing with the young man in the background who repeatedly told him to calm down and stop talking about hurting people. Thankfully, he didn't make it to our clinic. He was arrested on route by police who had set up a block on the road leading to our clinic.

He had multiple loaded guns in his front seat.

After we received news of the man's arrest, I successfully transferred my elderly man with suspected food poisoning to the local hospital for a CT and observation. I checked into the hotel my company booked for me, and I called our corporate overlords, begging them to close the clinic the next day for a staff meeting and debriefing. Not only did they tell me that wasn't going to happen, but they also advised me that, if I to fail to show up for my next shift in twelve hours at that site, I wouldn't be paid, my hotel wouldn't be covered for the night, and, if they did have to close, none of the staff would be paid.

I didn't sleep that night.

I also didn't eat much because, with my waning gastric abilities, with this level of stress, I simply couldn't physically do it. I drank a protein drink, and nibbled some crackers, took my medicine, and stared at the hotel popcorn ceiling for hours until the sun peered through the curtains.

The next day, it was a different slate of support staff, and they all arrived smiling, one by blissful one. My eyes were dark, my back hunched, and my body sweaty, and we hadn't even unlocked the door yet. Someone asked what was wrong. I told them. They reacted emotionally.

"No one told us!"

"I wouldn't have come into work today if I had known!"

"What the actual fuck?!"

"Corporate told me to stop being so dramatic," I said quietly.

I've lost count of how many times people in authority have told me I'm being dramatic.

It is *never* appropriate to tell someone they are being dramatic when they say, "I don't feel safe."

I repeatedly appealed to my regional manager for some kind of professional support over the next several months. I explained I started having nightmares about the would-be-shooters and it was affecting my personal and professional lives. It didn't help that each morning when I clocked into work, I was greeted with a police car stationed outside our urban clinic for several weeks while he was on bail.

The police presence didn't comfort me.

It reminded me that we were in active danger. That it was the holiday season and desperate people do desperate things. That the holidays were a time of high financial and emotional stressors, and this man might just have enough motivation to return to make good on his threat, but this time he wouldn't call us first to let us know he was coming.

The police presence reminded me I said no, albeit indirectly, to the wrong man one too many times. My nocturnal tortures transformed themselves into various scenarios of "What If" he returned. What if he came back to kill us? What if I never saw my husband again? "What if" can spiral into so many directions you're left spinning the moment you open your eyes. Eventually, I decided to go up the corporate rung, beyond my regional manager, to ask for help.

The Corporate Head I spoke to clicked her tongue disapprovingly when I asked her if the company covered counseling as a workers' compensation claim, and if I could start the process. "No, why would we? You're the only one having problems."

I couldn't sleep. I couldn't eat. I couldn't feel anything anymore.

All I could do was clock in and out and pray I stayed safe for just one more day, but no one was really listening to me.

How to Lose 100 Pounds

I wanted my corporate overlords to find my body.

Everyone had left the clinic a few moments earlier, but I lingered behind at my computer, using the excuse that I needed to close a few charts. Everyone was eager to leave, and no one hesitated. I was left alone in the dark as they set the lobby alarm.

At the age of thirty-two, I weighed myself one last time in the clinic, before closing the provider office door. With clothes on, the scale tipped to one-hundred-thirty-four, and I realized I lost nearly one hundred pounds, and I did it eating almost nothing but gelato for the entire year prior.

Earlier in that week, I met with my gastroenterologist, who threw his hands up in confusion, admitting that he didn't know the cause of my weight loss. He suggested it was stress related and we commiserated about the state of medicine after I told him about the two disgruntled male patients who threatened violence. I agreed stress played a role but I countered there had to be an underlying pathology because my stomach symptoms started before the work traumas.

It wasn't diabetes, which was the most common cause of gastroparesis.

It wasn't multiple sclerosis, which was a less common cause of gastroparesis.

It wasn't anything at all, according to him. It was normal to lose your appetite when your stress level was high and he argued that working in medicine in general was a recipe for unprocessed stress. Again, he wondered if my lack of sleep was contributing to my symptoms and suggested it might just be psychosomatic after all.

It wasn't normal.

No one was listening.

I pushed for a CT scan, I pushed for more of a workup, I pushed for him to keep going. He offered me an international prescription for a medication not approved in the United States, and looked at me disapprovingly when I told him I didn't want an experimental drug without a clear pathology. In medicine, you can't effectively treat what you don't know and the shotgun approach of throwing medications at a patient isn't something I ever appreciated.

He finished our last visit by stating my physical appearance wasn't improving due to the weight loss anymore, "You know, it's not a good look to lose that much."

I had no words.

"If you lose anymore, we're looking at a feeding tube." He closed my chart, stood up, and motioned for me to go to reception to make a follow up for three months.

At my highest, I was two-hundred-twenty-two so, part of me appreciated the weight loss. At first, I thought it was great. I welcomed the easy loss of pounds for the first time in my life with a bit of a smirk.

Be careful what you wish for, indeed.

Ten pounds gone seemed like a nice consolation prize for the worsening heartburn. Twenty pounds seemed like a fair exchange for the reflux that was now claiming my nights. When I hit thirty pounds lost, and my safe foods fell away one by one, I started to really worry. Forty pounds, and I began to panic when none of my physicians felt like it mattered.

I was fat before, and I was still clinically obese, so what was the problem?

Meanwhile, I faded. I faded away from fresh fruits and vegetables, unable to handle the fiber or the space they took up in my ischemic stomach. I faded away from meat, only able to handle bites of fish every few days. I faded away from anything and everything unless it was highly processed and could be rendered into a liquid in the safety of my mouth before being swallowed one painful bite at a time.

It was like swallowing knives. Carbonated knives.

They would dance in my stomach, jabbing me until I was bent over the sink, begging for deliverance from my pain, swearing I would never eat solid food again.

Just up the street from our apartment, an ice cream enthusiast returned from Italy brimming with the sacred knowledge of transforming food into gelato. I credit his cantaloupe, avocado, and cannoli gelato paired with the right sativa for helping me gain weight and survive the worst of my flares. Many of my coworkers laughed and said they wished they could eat infinite ice cream without their waistline expanding. They wanted to know my secret recipe. I even joked with the shop owner often that so many people told me they would die to lose weight if they could eat unlimited amounts of gelato, but there I was actually dying. I'm not sure if he ever realized just how dead serious I was.

It was only a matter of time before I gave up.

I had no support at work, and I was expected to keep caring for others as my body shut down and my mental state grew increasingly paranoid about aggressive patients. I had no support from my medical team and they all but abandoned a differential diagnosis for a cocktail of non-evidence based interventions. I had support from my husband, but he had transformed into a caregiver and was no longer a partner or a lover, but rather someone who cleaned up my messes.

I had finished my transformation into a zombie and was done with slowly rotting from the inside out. If I couldn't taste life, then I would taste the sharp kiss of decay on my own terms. I would take back control.

Back at the present moment, the moment I decided to kill myself, the clinic was quiet.

There was a soft glow from the computer, and I turned the light on. I didn't want to do this in the dark. I did want them to find my body. I wanted them to realize that they pushed me into this position, and that they failed one of their own. I wanted people to realize I was hurting, and my job was part of the reason I couldn't keep going.

I wanted my story to end in a cautionary tale.

I wanted my story to matter and I wanted to leave a mark that couldn't be so easily dismissed.

I opened my black medical bag, and I took out a bottle of Tylenol and my prescription of Xanax. The bottle of Tylenol was liquid because I knew my stomach struggled to handle anything, so pills were difficult even on good days. Today was most definitely not a good day. It was clear and unflavored, or so I thought, but it actually contained a cherry component I wasn't expecting. It was sickly sweet. I didn't want the last thing I tasted in this life to be so medicinal, but I had whole milk to help keep me from tossing it up too soon.

I lined up the Xanax in front of the black bag, and I took one. I waited a few moments.

I put the Tylenol to my lips. I gagged it down.

I breathed in through my nose and took another Xanax.

I counted the milligrams in my mind. I swallowed a sip of whole milk, trying to calm my screaming stomach, but only gagging more when the result was a burp that contained a cherry milkshake vibe. It was when I was trying to take the second gulp of Tylenol that a thought floated through my mind, fully formed and out of the darkness:

Gastroparesis results in delayed gastric absorption.

The clinician in me was speaking to the patient in me. Reminding me that the condition that brought me to the brink wouldn't let me successfully take the leap, at least not with an overdose where it relied on the stomach to perform. Calm, cool, and collected, Clinician Kateland continued out of the darkness:

Suicide attempts by oral ingestion with gastroparesis have a low success rate and will result in admission into an inpatient psychiatric unit after medical stabilization in an emergency setting.

Before I could formulate a response, either in real time or out loud, another voice, a different one, quietly but firmly suggested:

Think about your niece. It's not fair to leave her when she's only just getting here.

My sister was preparing to welcome her first child and we all knew she was going to need cardiac surgery upon arrival. I was pessimistic, and feared the worst prognosis. I chose not to have children for so many reasons, and one of the big ones was not wanting to condemn someone to a life like mine...

But what if she surprised me?

What if she surprised us all?

It wasn't fair to my sister, and it wasn't fair to her unborn daughter for me to leave just yet. I needed to make sure she got through her surgery and, if she did survive, I couldn't leave her without an example of what happens next to miracle children. Trembling, I picked up each pill and put them back into the orange bottle. I capped the Tylenol and drank the rest of the milk to counteract the sedative that was coursing through my veins. I drove home to my husband and didn't say a word about it.

A few days later, I asked for help.

Life During Diagnosis

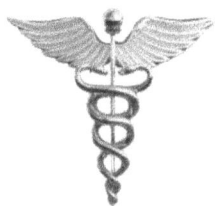

Meeting Your Maker

I met one of my healthcare heroes one month after I tried to kill myself at work.

The summer before, I purchased a ticket to a medical conference to see this hero speak as the keynote address. Dr. Zubin Damania spoke extensively about the dangers of moral injury in medicine and because I was so close to becoming a casualty of the system, I felt I owed it to myself to go to the conference.

Dr. Damania is a USCF/Stanford trained hospitalist who began a shadow career under the pseudonym ZDoggMD performing medical comedy, sketches, and songs à la Weird Al Yankovic. He combines medical training with honesty and words that connect with patients and providers alike. As I had been writing under my pseudonym, The Write Assistant, I wondered if I could bridge the gap between medicine and art, as well.

I considered him to be a digital mentor. I tuned in weekly for his medical rounds and participated in his paid Tribe for a time on social media. As I lost my white collar and my income, though, I couldn't keep paying the monthly fee to be a part of his exclusive online community– yet I enjoyed the videos and public community.

Two years before my suicide attempt, Dr. Damania posted a video to YouTube called "Say Something (We Won't Give Up On You)".

The audience is then taken for an emotional, lyrical, visual, and medical ride as the song is juxtaposed with images of clinicians being assaulted. The images and the song give way to real distress calls recorded on the job. The opening sequence of cries always gets me teary, but I listened to this video on repeat hundreds of times when I was at the bottom of my hole. There are three key moments in the video in which a black screen shows the following statistics:

0:36 minutes:

95% of healthcare workers report being physically or verbally assaulted.

1:10 minutes:

75% of all workplace assaults happen in healthcare settings.

2:22 minutes:

80% of emergency medical workers will experience violence during their careers.

He used the hashtag #silentnomore to encourage healthcare workers to speak up and, when those stories started to unfold, I slowly realized I wasn't alone. There were nights I spent playing this video on repeat. Those were the nights I stared at the razors too afraid to feel the slice of epidermis, and the nights I considered Tylenol cocktails. His lyrics and his advocacy are one of the biggest reasons I'm still here. He held a light up to the darkness that is mental distress in clinicians and gave me the language to ask for help.

The morning of the conference, I was nervous, both to meet my mentor and also to mingle with medical colleagues. I always struggled with networking within white collar settings because I didn't really know what to say and when, so I just politely mimicked the people around me. This time, though, I knew I wanted to meet him.

I needed to thank him.

To be fair, I was still actively suicidal. I was a little disappointed to wake up each morning because it meant I was only minutes away from toilet time (AKA torture time). I was desperate to find a reason to keep living and this conference, with its call to compassion and community, stirred something within my darkened soul: hope.

I got there early and picked a table right up front and center.

One by one, the conference attendees started to filter in, and I wasn't surprised to find the room booked solid. The gentleman to the left of me made small talk, asking where I practiced. I stumbled over the script I prepared for myself, that I was on a break to help my sister welcome her medically fragile first born into the world. We were focusing on family and health during my sabbatical, I assured him, and that fit right in with the theme of the conference. When I told him I was writing a book compiling my experiences in medicine, he nodded his approval. He didn't ask what the title was though and I was grateful he didn't push me for details I didn't have.

He confided in me, "I hate speaking first."

"Oh?"

"Yeah, I never get past the nerves."

My eyes narrowed as I read the name tags of the clinicians and thought leaders sitting at my table.

Oh my god, I'm at the speaker's table. I panicked internally.

Dr. Damania entered the room and took a direct line to his table. The one I just happened to be sitting at with the rest of the conference speakers. The people that you study under and are influenced by are more than just your mentors; they are your makers. They shape the way you see and interpret the world, and you apply their suggestions to your life. I am grateful for a voice like Dr. Damania, who made me realize there is life after trauma. There is hope after moral injury.

There are other ways to live your life, but you have to be willing to lose it all. The golden handcuffs keep all of us in our gilded cages, but only when we put our own health first can we take care of others appropriately. After he finished his talk, which was a combination of inspirational splices from his various talks online and an impromptu Doc Vader impression, he returned to our table.

Conference goers were already lining up at our table to speak to him.

Before he could turn to them, I got his attention from across the table, standing and offering my hand to shake his. "It's a pleasure to meet you, I just wanted to say thank you," I said.

He shook my hand and took a few pictures with me, my face betraying the excitement of meeting him in person.

"I, um, I'm taking a break from medicine right now. Your videos are one of the reasons I uh, decided to take a break instead of the other alternative." I teared up a bit, but I hoped I hid it well as I choked out an awkward, "Thank you."

"Walking away is sometimes the best choice you can make for yourself." He pulled me in for a big hug and I let go of the shame I had been carrying.

There was a type of absolution in that moment, it's when I admitted my darkest shame to a doctor I admired and he didn't look at me with pity or disgust, he looked at me with compassion other physicians lacked. With this small spark of kindness and creativity, Dr. Damania showed me there was still hope in medicine and I knew I couldn't give up because my story wasn't over yet.

Crossroad

"I don't know if this is really the right place for me."

I tried not to make eye contact with the director of the intensive outpatient program (IOP). My husband and I were sitting in his office and I was trying to convince myself that I didn't need this type of handholding.

The director tilted his head to the side and looked at my husband and then back at me. "You're at a crossroad. You're here for a reason and only you can decide if you want to keep going, but I think you should," the director replied.

I nodded weakly; he was right. I was at a crossroad: live or die.

He continued to talk about how their program required participants to sign a contract to attend therapy five days a week from 8 AM to 12 PM, complete nightly homework, and work with their psychiatrist to fine-tune a medicine regimen that optimized their mental health. It was a combination of dialectical behavior therapy, art therapy, and medication management, and my chief complaint indicated I was exactly where I needed to be:

Suicidal Ideation; failed attempt within the last three months

The contract devastated me at first, because it clearly stated no use of alcohol or recreational drugs. In parenthesis it included marijuana. At that point, my gastroenterologist had no recommendations for me beyond scaring me into eating more. He cautioned I was only a few pounds away from a feeding tube, but offered no referrals for second opinions and no real interventions. Marijuana was the only thing that kept the pain at bay and, even then, it did a subpar job at times. I cried wondering how I would survive the sensations germinating from my abdomen while also facing the demons of my mind.

One week into the program, I broke down in one of the therapists' private offices, telling her I felt like a disgusting drug addict who just wanted to die. It was at that moment when the therapist looked me up and down, took pity in my plight, and divulged a little bit of her story. This was her practicing compassionate healing in a way I could understand: she was telling me her story so I could see there were other endings available.

She shared with me that she was always drawn to medicine, but not as a medical doctor. She wanted to practice compassionate care as a therapist but that paid significantly less than being a doctor or marrying one as her family encouraged her to do. I snorted out loud when I thought of my Oma and mother joking about a similar situation for myself. Likewise, when I did finally settle on medicine, I never wanted to specialize in the high-paying fields. I was more interested in holding a hand out to the Zebras like me; I knew it was the frontlines that needed compassionate diagnosticians.

That day I tearfully contracted for my safety and agreed I wouldn't engage in self-mutilation or another suicide attempt while under her care.

I was still suicidal, but it was a function of the pain I was in. The therapist granted me an exception for the medical marijuana, acknowledging the contract was in place to keep patients clear headed. I wasn't clear headed when I was passing out on the bathroom floor in pain. If the medication made me functional, I wasn't an addict, she reasoned.

As I puffed on the dried flower each morning, a few hours before sessions started, I felt the fire in my belly receding slightly. It was just enough to keep a few crackers down, a few sips of whole milk, and the lifesaving omeprazole, but by the time my husband dropped me off at therapy, I'd be stone-cold sober and ready to face those demons with a circle of witnesses.

Each morning, we would open the session with a meditation. I liked that.

I had been practicing yoga since middle school, and I found great comfort in practicing even chair yoga in this setting.

The other participants had significantly ranged reactions from abject enthusiasm to downright disdain. The majority of patients were female with only two males matriculating through the program during my three months there. I started the program shortly after Thanksgiving and graduated the week of Valentine's Day. Four weeks before I matriculated into the program, my niece was born and she successfully surprised us all.

She survived.

She not only survived, but she thrived. She had a feeding tube placed after her emergency cardiac surgery at seven days old that damaged her vocal cords, but the doctors were amazed at her recovery. The day before I met her, the feeding tube was removed and, when I held her in my arms, I knew I needed to stick around and I promised her as much.

I just didn't know how I was going to make good on my promises yet.

So, each morning when the tall pixie-looking art therapist started our sessions with a mini-meditation, I felt relief, because I had long enjoyed yoga and a private meditation practice. She would pass around a basket filled with shells, stones, and feathers and told us to pick one during each meditation. If we couldn't focus on a word or mantra, she asked us to focus on the textures in our hands to take us up and away from our emotions. To ground us and remind us that we are more than the fleeting thoughts in our heads; we can use the world around us to redirect sensations in a healthier and happier way.

I enjoyed the stones, smooth and cold in my hands, and I nearly laughed as the ridges of the shells tickled my palms unexpectedly. I wasn't used to experiencing the world in a pleasurable way through my body anymore.

It was the morning we all had a Hershey's kiss that I collapsed outside the group session, in the hallway between the lobby and the bathroom. The art therapist handed each of us a tin foil-wrapped treasure and led us through a sensory meditation focusing on the melting chocolate on our tongue. We were instructed to let it melt and to avoid chewing, to swallow with purpose, and to redirect our thoughts back to the pure pleasure that is the indulgence of eating chocolate for breakfast.

Except for me it was an exercise in illness.

I ate so much chocolate I was literally sick of it.

I also didn't have any marijuana in my system, and I left my Zofran at home. When the first wave of nausea hit me, I had nothing to reach for in relief. I opened my eyes, frantically wondering if any of the other patients struggled with the morning meditation.

Nope, just me.

I bolted out of the room, retching into my hands. The bathroom was locked and I forced myself to swallow the vomitus while I waited for the sanctuary of the stall to open up for me. I spent at least twenty minutes crying in the bathroom, praying for some kind of relief from this purgatory. When I opened the door, one of the therapists was waiting for me.

She escorted me into a private room, and we conducted an episode evaluation for what they called a "dysregulated episode".

After that day, I started to open up in the circle. I shared that I was actually a physician assistant, or at least I had been, before I decided I wanted to give up my ghost after a shift. I spoke about my suicidal ideation in a detached, clinical way that the other patients lacked. They were much more emotional about their stories, and I realized that each one of us was a victim of our circumstances more than anything else. We were all inherently good people dealing with extraordinarily insurmountable circumstances.

The art therapist quickly became my favorite out of all the clinicians. It had been years since I felt as if I had permission to simply play, despite my husband trying to encourage me to find this freedom for years. I needed permission from someone professional, not someone who loved me. When she invited us to create collages, I found myself breaking through the worst of my moral injury.

I created a juxtaposed set of postcards in which a clinician in a white coat was floating away in a field, with mountains in the background. Jumbled text warned the viewer that "there is no cure," and in the background, a papier-mâché death mask laughed. The other postcard showcased a field of flowers and a bright blue sky, but there was no way for the clinician to cross the divide. It was the first time I truly experimented with putting my thoughts to visual expression. For years as a child, I compared my artistic talents to my sisters and those around me, judging myself as inferior. I realized I could combine images with my words to create powerful statements that resonated not only with me, but with the very fractured friends I was making in therapy, as well.

We were all desperate for someone to listen, and we all wanted new ways to communicate. Dialectical behavior therapy, along with applied art and music therapy, helped me say one unexpected day, "I don't think I want to die anymore. I'm not sure what I have to live for, but I don't think I want to kill myself."

The circle clapped.

Once I verbalized that I wanted to live, my therapist asked me who I was before medicine. She asked me to draw a portrait of myself and whatever came out onto the paper was who I was before the trauma. To inspire myself, I wandered the galleries of the city, taking in the sculptures and the paintings of the tortured artists around me. I realized, slowly but surely, that all of us had stories to tell but words sometimes escaped us.

I decided I was a turtle: a wise but snappish creature on which the whole world rested. It was time for me to return to my shell for a time to rest and to heal.

This turtle still had bills to pay, and while my husband was working full time, the income to living expense ratio was no longer in our favor once I gave up my white collar. Our bills were increasing, and our credit score was plummeting, but we were just trying to survive to the next day.

To help pay the rent, I took a job in the warehouse beneath my husband's retail job. I went from a white collar with golden handcuffs to a blue-collar packing job, but I was the happiest I had been in a long time. That job was situated right downtown, which meant I could see the lake on my lunch breaks, walk through the art galleries after work, and best of all: no one was going to die on shift!

The Giantess, Me

I fell in love with a giantess, one late autumn afternoon.

For the first time in my working career, my new blue collar job offered a mandatory thirty-minute lunch break. The irony, of course, was I couldn't eat. So, I used it to wander. I spent so many days inside clinics, under fluorescent lights and masked under layers of personal protective equipment and this was what I was missing. I was missing the sparkling diamonds that reveal themselves when the sun catches water at just the right angle. I was missing the sensation of sunlight on my skin as I explored the city. Slowly, I was starting to feel pleasure in a body that was still wracked with pain, and that made all the difference.

I truly believe that art is magic and magic saves lives. Art was a large part of my journey to Life 2.0, and it started on those daily walks.

So as my eyes scanned every inch of the life-size canvas collages of the giantesses, I felt an immediate connection to the artist. Three canvases were displayed behind the register of my favorite gallery downtown. In the center was Misoo Bang, the artist, and she was flanked by two other women she had illustrated in larger-than-life details. All three portraits were approximately five feet tall, and depicted women painted over collages crushing little people, cartoons, and institutions beneath their fearsome feet. They were huge. They were strong. They were staring the viewer down as if challenging them to come closer while also warning them they were not in the mood. Not today and not ever.

Those women radiated confidence and, at my lowest point, I wondered if I would ever find my own fearsome feet again.

I picked up one of the prints and read what the artist had to say about these larger-than-life-ladies:

The Giantess, a mythical woman of great size and exceptional strength, exercises self-agency and total control by the very nature of her physicality. Her form is central to the places created in "The Giantess" series where she occupies the largest space in every painting. The canvas is her territory – her own world – where she benevolently rules over a bastion of humans. Men who kneel beneath her. Composed of political and religious leaders, the male crowd clamors for dominance to the utter disinterest of the Giantess, whose concern, if she has one, is accidentally crushing a couple of tiny malefactors under one of her massive feet.

Outwardly, the series references a transformative, cultural response to patriarchy and male dominance by reversing the male-female power dynamic through physical size. Inwardly, however, it is a therapeutic intervention aimed at the women who modeled for the paintings, all of whom had been personally traumatized by male violence at some point in their lives.

The models are real women, just like those in our own community. They are colleagues, neighbors, and friends who, by entrusting their trauma to me, provided me with source material from which to depict each one reborn as a Giantess, free of her painful memories and

208

post-traumatic suffering. In the Giantess form, female power, self-esteem, and agency have been restored. In fact, the sense of power has grown to legendary, "superpower" proportions.

The series encourages women to make no apologies about physically dominating men. The Giantess does not seek revenge; rather, her purpose is to provide a release from the realities of gender-based violence and, however momentarily, imagine the freedom of a world devoid of hurtful memories and fear.

I couldn't hide the tears, and I tucked around one of the display corners to compose myself. Looking through my purse, I had enough cash to purchase it, so that day I decided to forgo even a liquid lunch and instead spent it on the Giantess that looked the most like me. None of them looked exactly like me, but I was trying to decide who I wanted to be next, and the one I chose looked confident.

Maybe this giantess could help me figure out how to be confident too. As I paid the cashier, I complimented the series, "They are awesome. Beyond words."

He informed me that the artist I was admiring worked shifts at the gallery and, if I came by often, I'd eventually bump into her. I paled at the thought. She was, in my estimation, a very successful artist with a prominent spot in a coveted gallery in the city. So, the idea of talking to her when I barely had a voice was too intimidating. I thanked him and said I'd keep an eye out.

I tucked the Giantess into my IOP folder, so each morning when I'd open it, I'd see her confident gaze holding mine, reminding me there is life after trauma. That men and their machines can't take everything from you. I didn't entirely believe her, but I desperately wanted to, so when the morning meditations were taste based, I pulled out my Giantess and focused on her eyes.

I didn't run crying to the bathroom again.

I started imagining myself as a Giantess, my own fearsome feet squishing an urgent care beneath me, tiny people streaming out not entirely in the nick of time. It was gruesome, yes, but that gruesome energy was no longer being directed toward myself.

Each day, after the morning meditation, the circle would be opened up for general discussion and check-ins. The therapist would go around the room and offer each person five minutes to talk. I slowly realized that each and every one of us was a victim of our circumstances.

In our private sessions, my therapist cautioned me against diagnosing or managing any of the others in my head. I admitted with a smile that their stories were what interested me, and it made me realize my life wasn't so bad. After all, I had a husband who was still standing by me (though our relationship was barely holding on), and, for the time being, we were renting a room in a shared house in the countryside that we could afford. My favorite part about that rental was that it was close to a nature museum. I would wander their grounds, reconnecting with nature, and admire the hand-carved wooden replicas of species I'd never seen before.

My therapist noticed how much I brightened when talking about art and creative endeavors and she suggested I start writing for pleasure again, in addition to the collage and line sketches.

I pushed back: I didn't know what I would write.

I hadn't written for fun in nearly ten years, not since I graduated with my bachelor's degree, really. I did have a successful copywriting business and pen name under The Write Assistant but I didn't know what it would look like to start writing for fun again.

One day, during the session, it hit me like a tidal wave. I was coloring one of my self-portraits while another group member shared memories of her alcoholic mother, and I realized how many of us just wanted someone to listen to our story. I could listen. I enjoyed listening. In fact, I had been listening all along. I started sketching out ideas in one of my journals about some of my favorite patient encounters over the years. My go-to stories when people ask me about what it's like working in medicine. The ones that made people snort with laughter or squirm with disgust; those were the stories that were interesting.

I wanted to write about the stories where I listened, and something interesting happened.

I wanted to draw and color and write.

I wanted to stand on my own two fearsome feet again.

In our one-room apartment, my husband had put up a white board and, when I got home, I created my first word cloud in years:

Zebra Stampede
Secular prayers of urgent care
Jean and her broken heart
Brooke and her broken heart
We are the broken-hearted warriors

Hypotheticals happen
We deserve dignity

There were more squiggles than syllables, but those dry erase marked words became the kernel of this book: The Secular Prayers of Medicine. I tried to show my husband the white board, eyes probably wide and less-than-sane appearing, but he shrugged weakly and hunched back over his computer. He didn't see the path I saw to my book and, ultimately, to my future, but I did.

At the same time, I started processing these memories, I entered a line drawing of birds fleeing a cityscape for that nature museum's annual call for artists. A few weeks went by, and I assumed my piece didn't make the cut but I was proud I participated. I was starting to participate in life again; I was peeking my head out of my shell and starting to connect with the people around me.

Occasionally, during my breaks at the retail shop, I'd run into some homeless people on the streets. Some of them preferred to think of themselves as nomads but, regardless, they weren't always entirely welcomed in the retail stores. Part of that had to do with smell and scaring off the tourists and part of that had to do with occasional shoplifting. I had befriended a few of the local nomads because, with my inability to smell, I could talk to them and assist them in finding low-priced gear without wrinkling my nose in disgust.

Basically, I treated them like human beings and not as inconveniences.

One day, during a lunch break, one of the gentlemen of the streets I helped earlier with a backpack was outside our door fiddling with a sling for a similarly disheveled woman. It was clear she broke her wrist based on the cast, and neither of them knew how to readjust the sling once she put her winter coat on.

"Need some help?" I offered.

As we struggled to get her arm in place, she admitted she was just discharged from the hospital with nothing for the pain. Pain is a common concern, and this is where the intersection of economics, race, and healthcare access come crashing down on the average person. Addiction is only a few pills away. I asked her if she had any papers from the hospital, but she grunted, saying they did her no good; she couldn't read them.

I read them for her. I explained how to take Tylenol and ibuprofen over the counter for the pain and, as I did so, I immediately realized she couldn't afford to buy them. I counseled her friend to keep her close, and I went next door to the pharmacy and bought all of us some snacks, drinks, and two bottles of medicine. Her gentleman friend thanked me again and told me that he'd watch my back on the streets. This instance of street medicine was the first time I "practiced" since putting my stethoscope in its box and I felt a familiar stirring within my soul.

As the city got increasingly dangerous, his friendship proved helpful as I knew he would often watch me as I walked to and from my job. By all accounts, he was a man I was conditioned to be afraid of my entire life: He was the scary "other." But he wasn't scary and he wasn't any different than me. He was the first man who showed me that sometimes strangers can be safe and that I still genuinely enjoyed helping people through healing.

As I drew close to my graduation from IOP, the week of Valentine's Day, I wondered if I would ever be "normal." My therapist and I started to unpack some of my sensory issues, and I was becoming more honest with her in our solo sessions about my nightmares. We revisited the Aspergers diagnosis, and she gently informed me Aspergers was no longer an accepted term because it referred to the Nazi doctor who experimented on Holocaust victims.

As I processed the way I viewed the world, I waded deeper and deeper into art as a means for community engagement. I started with our circle of sad patients. During group sessions, I sketched a cartoon bouquet of three spoons that looked like daisies. It represented "Spoonies," and how we all have a finite amount of energy to give. On the back of each heart-shaped Valentine was an inscription that read:

This Valentine Isn't Perfect and Neither are You and That's Beautiful.
Everyone deserves love.
Happy Valentine's Day.

The Valentines were laminated and included instructions to follow a hashtag, which took them to my social media channels highlighting mental health awareness, and specifically suicidal ideation, during Valentine's Day. I handcrafted 200 Valentines and offered them up to the group:

"If you'd like to participate, I've created 200 Valentines that are to be hidden throughout the downtown district, but you are free to hide them anywhere. I'll put them at the front registration next to the sign in sheet." I smiled shyly, holding up a Valentine.

"Yes!" one of the college students exclaimed. "I love treasure hunts and stuff, and I was getting so depressed about the holiday. I'm down."

She took ten.

The therapist encouraged me to pass around the stack I brought and, to my surprise, every single woman in the circle took a few; only the gentleman patient passed silently. About fifty were left at the front desk with the following invitation:

Valentine's Day is about more than just romantic love: It's about reclaiming self-love.

This Valentine's Day, if you are a dark heart touched by sadness, transform that into a random act of love by participating in the inaugural Broken-Hearted Valentine's Day installation in Burlington, Vermont. You can be a Dark Cupid by taking one, or many, of these laminated Valentines and hiding them in the downtown Burlington District the week leading up to Valentine's Day.

This guerrilla art installation is meant to inspire and remind us all that love is where we make it, and it's our imperfections that make us magic.

Collectively, my Dark Cupids and I peppered the downtown district with little love notes for ourselves, and for anyone who might chance upon them and we all felt, for a fleeting moment, a little more loved. I didn't realize that I was becoming an artist like the ones I idolized in the galleries simply by exploring my own creativity. A month after I graduated from the outpatient psychiatric program, the nature museum director reached out to let me know my line drawing was selected to be part of the exhibit. I was over the moon and I happily accepted, eagerly telling my family I was now an artist in Vermont.

I was becoming a real person, and then I became a giantess when I finally met Misoo. She was behind the register at the gallery one afternoon when I was taking my regular lunch break, and, even though I really didn't have the money, I picked up another Giantess and approached her at the register to purchase it.

"They are beautiful. I come here often to look at them," I started.

To my surprise, she was warm and appreciated the connection. Taking a chance, I admitted I reached out to her via Instagram a few months earlier and I wondered if she was still creating this series. She hadn't checked her messages in some time, but told me that she was.

"I think I'm ready to tell my story. I don't know if it's what you're looking for, though. I...I'm a clinician. A Physician Assistant, to be exact, but uh, I've stopped practicing to collect myself. I had two men threaten my life and uh, well, nothing really happened, but yeah."

My words trailed off and I inwardly cursed my awkwardness. Free-form speaking has never been my thing and, unless I had a social script already prepared, I was prone to stumbling, stuttering, and just generally picking the wrong words. It was an inconsistency that plagued me since childhood, and I hated it about myself. I was either on or I was so very off and, as I tried to connect with this artist I admired, I felt off. She surprised me again by asking for my information and a few weeks later, I was sitting on an oversized chair in her living room, and listening to her story.

She was born in the Bronx, New York, and then moved to Korea when she was only twelve months old. Her family remained there until she was eighteen before she returned to the United States to study art. She graduated from Florida Atlantic University and received a Master of Fine Arts in Painting in 2014 before moving to Burlington, Vermont. She was motivated by her dark childhood to explore what could never be said out loud through the power of pigment.

She was a survivor of childhood sexual assault.

As she shared her story, I thought of myself when I was her age, and I pushed the thoughts down. I was here to talk about my adult traumas, not childhood memories I had long since repressed.

But, as she described some of her symptoms as she grew older, I started to flashback to physician assistant school, and I remembered my lessons.

Childhood abuse is associated with depression, anxiety disorders, eating disorders, post-traumatic stress disorder, chronic pain syndromes, fibromyalgia, and irritable bowel syndrome. Childhood abuse survivors are more likely to engage in high-risk behavior, such as smoking, alcohol and drug use, and unsafe sex, to report overall lower health status, and to use more health services.

A variety of somatic symptoms are consistently higher in adults with a history of physical or sexual abuse compared to those without an abuse history. Women in primary care with a history of sexual abuse are often treated for psychosomatic complaints that manifest as:

Nightmares

Choking sensations

Frequent or severe headaches

Chronic genital or abdominal pain

Binge eating or self-induced vomiting episodes

I shook my head internally, trying to keep the medical jargon from pulling me away from her story. But her tale and her symptoms reminded me so much of my childhood that I couldn't stop thinking about it, even after we finished our session that day.

It was then my turn to speak.

I told her about my childhood illnesses and the doctors that didn't listen.

I told her about my desire to help others and to find the Zebras that were without a diagnosis or herd of their own.

I told her about how medicine was not at all what I thought it would be and, even though I was making good money, nothing could compare to how much I was hemorrhaging as a Zebra with an unclear diagnosis and even hazier prognosis. I told her about the two men and their guns, and how I was so scared they would come back any day. I told her about all my different nightmares. I dreamt about gunmen. I dreamt about being raped. I dreamt about my belly swelling with deformed fetuses and then exploding on an operating table. I dreamt about losing control of my body and my teeth shattering into the sink.

After we shared our stories, it was time to move past them, together, with paint. Misoo told me to change into a few of the outfits that I felt the most confident in; we'd model all of them to find the best fit.

I remember bringing my white coat, a blouse, and some slacks, but that didn't feel right. I also brought a comfortable skirt with a blue shirt as an homage to my writing persona, but that felt incomplete, too, so instead I stepped out wearing my red and white hibiscus dress first.

When she saw the flowing red dress dotted with white blooms, she said, "That's the one."

"Really? You don't want to see the others?" I asked.

She didn't.

I thought I needed to present myself as a professional white-collar authority, but that's not really me. I'm also not just a hippie without a cause; I'm a Robin Hood of Hospitals and my giantess is about crushing medical institutions that forgot that we should do no harm. I realized I had always been an artist, but I'd always suppressed that side of me, so that afternoon, as I connected with another soul who dared to share her past, I started to lean into the symbolism.

In my mind, my dress and my giantess represent the following concepts:

The white hibiscus represents purity and femininity and is part of the mallow family. Mallows are excellent for soothing nausea and are a staple in the gastroparesis world for taming wayward symptoms so to me the flowers represent the beauty in my pain. Finally, back in the old days, a doctor's coat splattered with blood was a sign they were a successful surgeon. I wanted my dress to represent an inversion of those colors, a reclaiming of the idea that violence makes a diagnosis. I told her I wanted the white flowers against a bloody background to represent the hope that there is life after diagnosis.

I gave up my story to her hands and told her that I trusted her implicitly. She cautioned me that some of the models had expressed frustration that their portrait wasn't what they thought it would be when she finished, but I reassured her I was here for the experience, not a product.

I was here because it was time for me to stand on my fearsome feet again.

The giantess, me, was transformed into a woman with a halo crafted from the ceilings of the Vatican and a throne of Notre Dame. No men scurried beneath my feet in the Holy City, and at first I was kissed with a flicker of disappointment. I wanted to crush the men. I wanted to see them squirm beneath me. But then I realized I wasn't a monster. Even though my body was more zombie than woman, I didn't need to lend myself to dark thoughts. I was loftier than that, with my head in the sky and my feet grounded in reality. The giantesses weren't seeking out to destroy the men, no, they were simply reclaiming what was always theirs, and if the men got in the way, that was their own foolish fault.

My giantess held domain over the very institutions of divinity and education, of medicine and of man, and I became more than I was before:

The giantess, Kateland, is the Patron Saint of Complicated Clinical Cases, Diagnostician to the Dismissed, Protector of the Physically Forsaken, and the Adopted Advocate Mother of Zebras. She is the clinician that listens and her gaze reminds the viewer that, when hypotheticals happen, we always deserve dignity.

I vowed one day to save up enough money to bring the Giantess, me, home, but not before she went on display with the other models. We were all transformed by Misoo's vision and, even though the world outside was raging with political unrest and viral catastrophe, I thought we were hanging on. Just as I started to stand on my own two fearsome feet, COVID-19 surged into a worsening reality and, as the world shut down, we ultimately lost our little spot in Vermont to circumstances beyond our control.

Ice Cream Conspiracy

By the time I had decided I wanted to give life another shot, my husband and I found ourselves in a position of homelessness. A local church had paid our last month's rent and a few medical bills, but we were barely scraping by, and each day the pandemic worsened just outside our doorstep. We were vulnerable and, in our time of need, I fell to my knees and begged my parents for help.

As I graduated from my IOP, my therapists warned me that there was more work yet to be done. Much needed to be uncovered about my childhood, and that would only happen when I was ready. Before I was ready to do that, though, I needed to get back to work.

It seems strange that I even considered returning to the frontlines as my colleagues were literally garbing themselves in garbage and I still hadn't found a diagnosis for my wasting syndrome. But, this time, instead of money, I was motivated by hope. As the pandemic raged on, our local Health Department put out a call for any clinical staff to help with testing and vaccinations.

It was time to dip my toes back into the world of medicine, but on a volunteer basis. I would return to my roots and remind myself why I waded into this world in the first place. As my niece continued to grow, surprising all of us after her successful heart reconstruction a mere seven days after her arrival, I continued in my resolve to make the world a safer place for her and all the other Zebras.

I answered the call and, a few weeks later, I was trained up and ready to start jabbing.

I use the term "jabbing" with a modicum of sarcasm. As one who focuses highly on words, I find the propagandization of phrases fascinating. I have no doubt that the early 2020s will be a controversial time in history which will be studied and picked apart for decades to come, but I was interested in the trends from the conspiracy theorists. They believed the vaccines were not divinely inspired by their Lord Trump, but rather a plot from Bill and Melinda Gates to further take over the world by injecting nanobots into our blood streams.

Among other variations.

People prone to believing these conspiracies started referring to the vaccine as "the jab" but in reality, this intervention saved millions of lives.

Stepping into my old community center, I was immediately greeted with memories of sweaty dodgeball with blue and yellow mesh vests. This was the place we learned to play but it was also the place we went to get our community vaccines when I was a kid. My left arm reflexively ached as the deltoid recalled my tetanus shot from so many years ago. When we were middle schoolers, we all lined up in the gymnasium and one by one, we got injected, not jabbed. We were vaccinated for the greater good and for our own good. Somehow in the 1990s, we understood the concept of herd immunity and civic duty more than we did three decades later.

Herd Immunity:

(Noun)

Resistance to the spread of an infectious disease within a population that is based on pre-existing immunity of a high proportion of individuals as a result of previous infection or vaccination.

The level of vaccination needed to achieve herd immunity varies by disease but ranges between 83 - 94% of the population.

Herd immunity is especially important to the 3% of the American population that Yale Medicine estimates to be moderately-to-severely immunocompromised. These are the people who truly cannot survive an infection and may not be able to handle a vaccine. It's not about imaginary preferences about which chemicals can enter your precious progeny; it's about keeping these people alive.

And that's where civic duty should come in:

Civic Duty:

(Noun)

Responsibilities of citizens to the general community.

Examples of civic duties central to American culture include voting, community volunteering, practicing tolerance, and staying informed.

The guidance counselor who taught us about safe sex kept us informed, and the women who volunteered to vaccinate us as children showed me what it meant to volunteer for the community. We learned about civic duty in these halls and yet so many of my peers forgot. They forgot that we had mandatory social studies that made us question discrimination and act in ways that uplifted the most vulnerable in our society as opposed to abandoning them.

One of my most concrete memories of volunteering early in my adolescence was sitting beside a dying woman with Alzheimer's. She was abandoned by her family in a nursing home and I was paid to be her sitter. Theoretically, I would read to her, assist her with meals, and just generally help her pass the time for a few hours each week, but it quickly became clear she had no interest in media, food was a bane to her, and she just wanted the sweet release of death.

Later in life, I recognized that desperation as an adult who craved my own sweet release.

My Alzheimer's patient was at peace only when in sleep, her frail body skeletal and wrapped in skin wispy as a spider's web. She had more than one foot in the grave, but it was the aides who kept grabbing her hand and ripping her back onto this plane of existence.

When I was there during her lunchtimes, she would ignore her mushy plate full of mashed potatoes and meat gravy. She would wail and spit the meager spoonfuls back at me, until I realized the one food she would eat, nay, relish, was the small cup of vanilla ice cream. I felt a childlike thrill as I consistently gave her the ice cream before trying to get her to take a few bites of the salty, savory mush piles left behind.

I only got away with that once or twice. When I realized what would happen if she didn't eat the food, I couldn't sleep for days.

Her mouth was turned upwards, and she was force-fed an En-sure.

She cried, begging the nurse to stop, her fully formed sentences choked with chocolate and ignored by a woman charged with her health.

I was a teenager, and I was her witness, but I couldn't do anything but listen.

She died a few weeks after I met her, but every chance I got I snuck her as many ice cream cups as I could. She thanked me after eating her ice cream and shook her head each time I offered her anything else. She pointed to the water when she wanted some, whereas before, she ignored it entirely. The lessons I learned at her deathbed remain with me today and, when I am faced with profound sorrow, I still remember the power of ice cream: a spoonful of sugar always helps the bitterness go down.

So, it only made sense to me, a few months into volunteering at the vaccine clinic, to suggest an ice cream truck for the first weekend of pediatric vaccines. The director loved my suggestion.

"Why not?" She flashed a bright smile. "I'm in charge of giving out food permits and I'm in charge of this."

Posters were put up throughout the town and a digital mockup was made advertising the complimentary sweets after each shot for the first day of pediatric vaccines. I was pretty pleased with myself, mostly because I was still on a near-liquid diet at that time, and the idea of getting free ice cream when we were collecting food stamps was too good to pass up. Until the comments started pouring in online.

"How SICK! They're bribing our kids with sweets!"

"Where's the ice cream for the adults? This is proof they are indoctrinating the children. We can't let this happen in our town!!"

The comments got progressively more aggressive, and I felt a flash of terror rise up in my throat. I didn't want to have another disgruntled patient come at me, and I realized the current political climate fostered gun violence more than ever. The comments started to get to me, but, because of my involvement in far too many social obligations to try to rebuild my life, I couldn't turn away.

I blocked them out while I was at the vaccine clinic and each day I grew more confident in my clinical skills. But each night the anxieties would return, and I was without a therapist even still because of our lack of funds. I was doing my best to employ my skills learned at IOP, but the more time I spent in my childhood home, the more my old childhood parasomnias started to bubble up. My husband told me the night terrors had returned and I was screaming in my sleep.

During the day though, my clinical voice returned. I focused on my work. I pinned a photograph of my niece and me squatting next to a pumpkin to show my patients who I was and why I was there. I wasn't part of some great conspiracy, and I certainly hadn't been employed or reimbursed by anyone for quite some time, so it wasn't money driven. No, I was driven by the hope that one day my niece would be able to come out and play dodge-ball or eat an ice cream at the new plastic playground with us. I was driven by the hope that my fellow Zebras wouldn't have to cower inside while the general public lamented how unfair it was their regularly scheduled haircuts were late.

"Go ahead, ask her," a mother implored her twelve-year-old son as he anxiously rolled up his sleeve.

"What's up?" I put my hands down to show him I had nothing sharp, and I wasn't going to surprise him with anything.

"Ok, um, yea." He gulped trying to find the words. "Are there 'bots in there?"

"Bots?"

His words were a jumble of pressured syllables, "A buncha-my-buddies-aren't-getting-it-cuz the robots. Their parents said there are little robots in there and that I'm stronger without them."

"That's a really good question," I started as he leaned in, surprised. "A lot of people have been saying that but I'm happy to tell you that's not true. I wouldn't do anything to a patient that I wouldn't do to myself. I can't wait to get my second shot so I can go play with my niece."

He beamed a bright smile at his mother and then asked if we could snap a shot while we did the deed. I said of course, but only if his mother would send me a copy. At that time, I had reinvented my online handle The Write Assistant and started writing under that name. I was rebuilding a life for myself right where I left it so many years ago, and I was committed to figuring out what went wrong before.

Little did I know I was only a photograph away from disintegrating into all the diagnoses I had been running away from and toward over the last thirty-four years.

Kit Kats and Blunts

"Can I have a Kit-Kat? I always get a Kit-Kat!" My voice was bright, loud, and clear in the way only a young child could be when whining for a treat. Again, I asked for candy, but the voice that was coming from inside my throat didn't match my thirty-four-year-old body.

The voice coming from inside me hadn't spoken in decades and she was hungry.

"She's, uh, she's having some kind of mental breakdown," my husband choked the words out, trying desperately to hold my hand and keep it, and me, from bouncing away from the emergency room receptionist.

"I'm here for a KIT-KAT! Kit-kat…kit…KAT."

"Go sit down." He sighed to keep from screaming, "Please."

"Okay."

I sat cross-legged on a green plastic chair, watching the ER lobby bustling with life. I stopped invoking the request for chocolate and settled in, knowing I was in exactly the right place. I was at the hospital, and I was going to get checked in to be seen as a patient.

This is the point in my story where I finally lost my mind. It happened when my memories decided to resurface, and my body couldn't keep up anymore. After decades of building walls and stories to hide the truth, the insanity came crashing out of me in one glorious meltdown after coming face to face with a picture of my childhood molester. Like a nut cracked open, my brain matter was spilling out of my head and into the world in the most unpredictable of ways. I found, in my humbling experience, that in order to have a true mental breakdown, I needed to commit to being committed.

I got out of the psych ward after seven days of insanity, but only because I gathered my fractured wits to follow the breadcrumbs home.

This story are those crumbs. One month before I finally confirmed my diagnosis of a vascular malformation, the one that had been eluding me for thirty-four years, I tipped into full-blown breakdown. I was tired, I was starved, I was dehydrated, and then I went mad. Some small part of me was still present. I kept blinking wildly as if I were attempting to shake off the sleepy surrealism of the world I found myself in all of a sudden. It was as if I was floating above the scene and watching a clinical case series of another patient, another person, as they demonstrated psychiatric manifestations. Words floated around in the pea soup of my sentience.

What do you see, Katie?
I see green…blue.
Kit…kat. Kat…Kit.
What do you see?

Green…
Blue…
Kit-Kat-Kit-Kat-Kit-Kat.
Green.

My husband stood next to me, protectively, trying to minimize my talking, shushing me gently but really lacking the words to navigate this situation. If I were in my right mind, I would have been mortified. Normally, when I walk into a medical office, I keep walking until I settle down in my office. I put on my white coat, or my scrubs, and I wait for the patients to be triaged and put into rooms for me to dissect. Normally, I'm the one ordering the Haldol and not experiencing it.

That day, though, I had fragmented into all the different versions of myself I had been cultivating over the decades, and I couldn't hold it together any longer. At that very moment, in the lobby, I was not Kateland Kelly, PA-C, but rather Katie Kelly, child actress, toddler, and Kit-Kat enthusiast.

You might recall that, back in the day, Katie, or rather I, was always praised for being a well-spoken and precocious child and for a few years flourished in front of the cameras. Whether I was on set selling national brands of cereal or overalls, I could cry on demand, I could memorize lines, and I had a smile with dimples that sold, sold, sold. But this version of me was decades in the past, or so I thought.

Now Katie came out to play, as did the others, after so many years hidden deep, deep inside me because she saw that photograph.

My husband had met Katie only a few hours earlier when I threw myself to the ground of my childhood home. The body absolutely keeps score and like a recorder, it remembers everything. My husband watched me as I flipped onto the ground, face down against the carpet as the memories of sexual assault flooded my brain. I screamed as I begged it to stop but I wasn't talking to my husband and he couldn't get through to me.

In his desperation, my husband whipped out his cell phone threatening to record me. He thought I was having a panic attack. He thought I was being dramatic. Usually, the threat of a camera recording "bad behavior" was enough to snap me to attention, but when my screams continued blatantly unconcerned about any type of observation, he knew I was gone, gone, gone.

Somehow, we got into the car.

Somehow, he drove me to the hospital in which I was born.

Somehow, I had the foresight to grab one of my journals and a package of markers, and I started writing while he drove.

Black ink met with red met with blue and all of a sudden, the stories started bubbling up. I wrote with frenzied hands repeating phrases. They were the keywords to remembering my assault but it was all jumbled. All I knew was that if I didn't write down what I could remember it would go back beneath the sands of time, bubbling beneath the surface until the next time the trauma decided it needed an audience.

This adventure took place in the summer but the hospital was still struggling to handle the influx of COVID-19 patients and all their complications. Cardiac cases had priority, as did bleeders, so it was no small surprise that I sat and waited in my stewing insanity for what seemed like hours. It certainly wasn't minutes. My husband guided me away from the triage window into the front lobby after a few seats opened up, relatively apart from other patients. Then again, it was packed, so I couldn't help but notice other patients as they noticed me.

Katie Kelly yawned. She was tired.

"This is freakin' ridiculous!"

A voice broke through the din and my senses sharpened until I focused on a young, white woman, dripping in frustration and privilege.

She continued, "I've been waiting here for *hours*. Literally hours. My stomach is, like, killing me and no one's doing anything."

She was sitting with her legs daintily crossed, toes tapping in frustration. She picked at her manicured hands while the partner in her conversation responded. I quickly triaged her in my head, my mind warping from the dramatic toddler to the seasoned clinician. Her voice was calm and measured, despite her words, and her position didn't indicate any pain.

She was stable.

"Yeah, no. I'm not going to wait until next week to see my doctor. They can take care of it now." She scoffed into her phone.

My eyes narrowed as I watched this woman, and I wondered if she was planted there. I wondered if *all* the patients were actually planted there for me to diagnose.

They're watching me. They're watching all of us.

Katie Kelly decided to take a nap and, with one quick flick of the switch into paranoia, I slipped into a delusion of observation as Kateland Kelly, PA-C, was absolutely convinced that not only was she, or rather I, being videotaped, but I was also there to break the cycle of abuse that was rooted in systemic racism, sexism, and xenophobia.

I was there to Save. Us. All.

I already decided the Connectikaren, my affectionate phrase for women who use their white-picket privileges to boss others around, was unworthy of my triaging skills. I turned away from her and looked to those seated to my left. They were a young Hispanic couple whispering urgently to each one another, the man asking her if she was OK.

She responded, in Spanish, that her stomach hurt.

She was scrunched up in a strange position, trying to tuck her legs underneath her to find some semblance of relief. I made eye contact with her. My husband squeezed my hand concerned that my crazy was going to come out and play with the other patient waiting.

It did.

"Hola. Mi nombre Kateland. Tienes dolor con tu estomago?" I asked her in broken Spanish if she had stomach pain.

"Si. Con Comida," She nodded slowly, responding, "Yes, with food."

"Dónde? Where?" I asked.

She pointed to her epigastric region, and I nodded, too; she hurt where and when I hurt. I understood and I knew her position wasn't going to give her much relief kinked up that way. I grabbed

234

a chair that was about fifteen feet away and dragged it back over to her. I pantomimed for her to untuck her legs and to put them up on the now-creatively arranged furniture to put her in a modified supine position.

Based on the way she was holding her stomach, I flitted through a differential diagnosis for epigastric pain in my mind, starting with the ones that could kill her first and then the ones that would just make her wish she was dead.

Pancreatic cancer
Mesenteric ischemia
Median arcuate ligament syndrome
Dissecting abdominal aortic aneurysm

She stretched her legs out and sighed, seemingly relieved just a touch. I wished I had some alcohol pads to offer her; she looked like she might vomit, and rubbing alcohol is as effective as Zofran (prescription nausea medication). Internally, I railed against the idea of this woman, who was obviously in pain, having to wait. She was a far cry from the young white woman complaining about the lack of service, and I felt the rising tide of social justice warrior.

I had to Save. Us. All.

Next to where the Connectikaren was still yapping away, an elderly black man struggled to pick up the lobby telephone while shuffling around on a wheelchair. He was trying to call for a ride home, but the way the telephone was set up, it was hard for him to reach it while bound to the chair. His right hand was shaped like a claw, perched close to the chest as if he were hiding a treasure deep within, while his left lacked the dexterity to grasp the handle. We were separated by close to twenty feet, but, when the telephone clattered down, not onto the floor but into the garbage, it took only a few seconds to realize no one was going to help this man.

Before my husband could stop me, I jumped out of my seat, closed the gap between us, and picked up the phone. The man looked up at me surprised, and I refused to hand it back to him until I had wiped it with a Sani-cloth.

"Do you need help dialing?" I asked in measured English. The bright tones of Katie Kelly were officially gone and replaced with the easy-going style I take when approaching a patient in acute pain.

He did need help.

After he made his call, he thanked me and tried to shuffle away but the wheelchair brake was held tight against the wheel and his right leg kept flopping out of the step.

Hemorrhagic ischemia?

"I had a stroke. Would you believe these fuckers just put me on the street! They didn't do *shit* for me."

His clawed hand and his floppy foot were both bare, the nails sharp, yellow, and dirty. I kneeled before him and placed his foot back in the step. It fell out again with a sickening thud. I put it back, but this time, I sat cross-legged on the floor next to him, ensuring it stayed put. I was ministering to the sick. Of course, I would plop down on the floor and distract him with small talk while waiting on his ride; he had just experienced a life-threatening event and was left with half of his functionality and no social support. Hospital staff dumped him in the lobby and figured transportation was his problem now, muscle weakness be damned.

As for the remainder of the patients in the lobby, how could they just scroll in bored silence when a fellow citizen needed assistance?

Kateland Kelly, PA-C, believed, and believes, in the importance of listening and acting in small ways. Medicine isn't magic, but kindness is, and sometimes taking a patient's hand, or foot, is the most powerful intervention there is. Still swirling within my own madness, a new thought danced behind my eyes:

Is he Jesus?

Was he waiting for me to let me know I'm in the right place?

Was he there to show me I was on the right track to saving myself?

I didn't have a basin in which to wash his feet in that lobby, but caring for him while my mind deteriorated was the closest thing I would get to divinity that week. I wasn't washing him, but I was empathizing with him and imagining how it would be to walk in his shoes, and it was powerful.

"All I want to do is go home and smoke a blunt. You feel me," the man in the wheelchair said.

"I feel you!" I laughed enthusiastically.

I think Jesus just offered me a blunt.

His ride came and he went. My husband asked if I would be OK by myself for a few minutes and I said I was. Following my lead, he helped wheel our newfound friend outside, forgetting I was a psych patient and should *not* be trusted. However, when he returned, I was sitting cross legged in my original chair once again, bouncing up and down, wondering if I could get a Kit-Kat before being admitted to the psych ward.

I just couldn't wait for someone to listen.

Seven Days of Insanity

The American healthcare system fails nowhere so spectacularly than with mental health. This is astoundingly true in mental health crises, and the only reason I am able to share my story is because of my medical degrees and awareness. Without those two tools, I would have been cast to the bottom of society to rot.

We need to do better.

We can't keep hurting people by stigmatizing mental health. Of course, I don't advocate tolerating verbal or physical abuse in any setting, but as clinicians we are responsible for investigating behavior and de-escalating crises to the best of our ability. Do no harm but take no shit, for the love of all that is holy.

I practically skipped my way to ER bay #3, eager to jump up on the bed and tell my story.

When a psychiatric patient is admitted to an ER, they are placed under strict observation. A patient care attendant, affectionately known as a "sitter" in the industry, keeps watch of their behavior. The sitter isn't usually medically trained beyond some basic hospital orientations, but they help remove the burden of care from the nursing staff. They are essential in documenting behavior as the patient cycles through their symptoms. As I jumped on the bed, actively fracturing, I was incredibly suspicious of my sitter.

They made me change out of my clothes and I protested when they took my prayer beads: my jade mala.

"You might hurt yourself."

My body was already blossoming with roses from where my fists battered, scratched, and rammed my body so their concerns were justified.

Gomez, the attendant I do remember, was somewhat polite, but he engaged in my fantasies by asking active questions which only worsened my paranoia. I sincerely believed that I needed to be admitted into the hospital because I was going to uncover the true pathology behind my body and I told him as much. In my delusions, I thought I was going to save myself and all the other people stuck on the psych ward, I just had to get there first.

As I explored my room with my wide eyes, the child version of me quickly flipped into a middle-aged white woman, dripping with disgust and privilege when I noticed my stretcher sheets were dirty. I was filled with indignant rage: How dare they be dirty! What type of hospital was this? I screamed at the "housekeeper" to keep my sheets clean, imitating the cruel, dismissive tones of the rich Connectikaren I noticed in the lobby.

Looking at Gomez with exasperation, I instructed him to write EVERYTHING DOWN, imagining him to be my personal scribe!

The hospital staff had taken away my markers and pens, you see, so I couldn't write anything down. I struggled to explain my symptoms verbally and, when the doctor finally came, she asked me what brought me in. I asked for paper and pens to write down what I was experiencing and this is what came out:

I struggle with verbal expression when overwhelmed.

And that, dear audience, is the complaint that landed me a seven-day stay in the very hospital I was born so many years prior. I can recognize it now for what it was: an autistic breakdown years in the making.

That first night in the emergency bay I had two distinct delusions while I was waiting for a bed to open up:

Paranoia:

The television was communicating with me. This I was absolutely certain, and it continued until the day I was released from the hospital. As the nurses explained, all the televisions were connected and, due to a glitch, occasionally flickered with static. There was no way to predict when the static would pop through, but in my delusion, I thought if I asked the TV a question and it flickered immediately after, the answer was "yes." It was clearly digital divination in my broken mind.

Grandeur/Observation:

I truly, sincerely believed I was part of a documentary that was going to expose all the child molesters in my region. I needed to get admitted not because I was unstable, but because I was going to help everyone.

Gomez continued to egg me on, or at least that's how I interpreted his banter while we waited for a bed on the unit upstairs. At this point, I had been awake for several days, and that is a sure sign of mania. As I shortly learned, one of the ways down from mania is with a quick shot in the ass of a sedative.

"I don't want to stay here anymore. I have things to do," I said, jumping up suddenly.

"You can't leave." Gomez didn't leave his chair.

"But I have to get started," I implored him, wondering if the producers of the documentary I was writing were waiting for me upstairs yet.

"You have to wait." He looked at the door, "But I can't stop you."

Some part of me floated within that pea soup of my sentience and wondered if he really said that out loud. Because if he did, that would have been wildly inappropriate.

"I need to be discovered," Katie Kelly, the child version of myself whispered quietly, eyes wide and searching for the best camera angle to catch my eyes.

Gomez leaned forward, and while I'm fairly certain he did not actually say this, I distinctly heard him say: "You've already been discovered."

Because that is precisely what gave me permission to perform my next feat of insanity. Like I said, you really have to commit to being committed. I bolted right out of my room before he could react and took a sharp left, to the screams of nursing staff. Suddenly, I had transformed from a rambling maniac into a roaming one, and that's a Code Grey. Code Grey is the most common code called in a hospital setting, and refers to an aggressive or dangerous patient or visitor on the loose. It means run and hide, or shelter in place; it also means grab the Haldol and get security on set.

I really did think I was *on set*.

As four nurses and one police officer tackled me to the ground, I complimented them on their realistic take down skills. Suddenly I was face up, back pinned to the ground as a Disney princess stared at me. She had a beautiful blonde braid, blue scrubs and snowflakes decorating her name badge which displayed "Elsa".

Let it go…let it go…

The royal nurse reassured me, "It's OK. You're OK. You're doing great."

Suddenly, the princess had a needle in her right hand. I screamed, loudly. I felt a pinch and clinician Kateland Kelly, PA-C warned the others that we were going to take a nap now. Then all of my raging personalities faded to black.

After an unknown amount of time, my eyes fluttered open. I was in a small, dark, and nearly empty cell lying flat on my back on a hard, rounded rectangular bed that took up most of the room. As I sat up, I noticed a single-serve vanilla ice cream, much like the ones I used to feed my dementia patient. I picked it up, curious about how and why it was put there, and set it back down because it had long since turned to liquid.

I gravitated toward the tiny square of light in the door – plastic crisscrossed with reinforced metal. Just inches from my pressed-up face, I watched another patient being brought back to their holding cell. In my mind, it was a scene of systemic racism and I flipped into a different personality: Social Justice Warrior Kate.

A small Black man stood next to a hospital cop. It was obvious he was confused and he looked incredibly frail. The hospital cop told him repeatedly to wash his hands with increasing agitation. The old man shook, and from my limited vantage point. it was obvious he was having difficulty operating the push bar and co-ordinating the soap dispenser. He had a slight tremor and I wondered if it was a side effect of medication or of an intrinsic pathology like Parkinson's.

BAM! BAM! BAM!

The hospital cop slammed his fist against my door three times in quick succession, startling me and the elderly man equally, "I said wash your hands old man!"

Before I could stop myself, Social Justice Warrior Kate yelled, "Hey! He doesn't understand you! Be nice!"

The cop focused his angry gaze on me and said, "If I wanted comments from the peanut gallery, I'd ask you. Shut up."

At the time of this exchange, our city had been the subject of investigation into systemic racism in our police department. As all the different stories were scrambled inside my mind at that moment, Social Justice Warrior Kate decided it was her duty to protect this marginalized man. Unfortunately, Katie Kelly was feeling particularly petulant and chimed in with a little bit of her juvenile antagonism.

"Why would you say something so politically explosive when the local department is under investigation for racism and assault?" I bounced up and down in my rounded cage, grinning foolishly as the words babbled out, mania on full display.

BAM!

"I said shut up. Keep talking and find out what happens." The hospital cop motioned to his partner to get the elderly man into his own cell and, before I knew it, both guards were in my room.

The hospital cop pushed me up against the wall, twisting my right breast violently in his palm, "This is what happens when you don't shut up. Do you want me to get the doctor? Huh?"

He twisted my breast harder, and his palm slipped, causing my shirt to twist under him. With an unexpected flip, I inverted myself and sprung away from him topless. His partner barely had a chance to react before I made it to the open cell door.

Screaming, I ran across the unit toward the nurses' station. I pounded my fists, topless, against the clear plastic protectors, "Help me, please help me. He's hurting me!"

They stared at me bug-eyed inside their fishbowl. They watched as the cops tackled me, forcing my face down on the floor. I immediately started convulsing; I didn't want to be face down. It brought back too many repressed memories, and I begged the nurses to keep me face up. No one listened as they carried me back into the padded cell, pushing me face down into the raised rectangle, it's purpose now perfectly clear:

It was the equivalent of an adult Circumstraint.

It had straps that came out on all four points, and along my abdomen, keeping me in place.

The hospital cop positioned himself toward my head and yelled at the nurses who entered the room, "This one's strong!"

"Damn fucking straight I am, you fucking PIG!" I yelled right back at him, inches from his face.

He slammed my head down and I felt wet in my hair.

Am I bleeding?!

I couldn't find the words as they tied me down, nor when they injected me once more that evening. As the sedatives rolled through my system, I realized no one was there to listen to me. There was something comforting about the way the straps held my wrists, and even as my body convulsed against the words that were bubbling up from my subconscious, I found myself surrendering to the darkness once again.

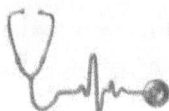

"Oh, honey, your hair is a mess!" A kind voice pierced through the light, suddenly flooding my consciousness.

I was alive, but where was I?

I sat up, groggy and uncertain, but before I could get a word out, the nurse offered a pill in a cup and cheerfully said, "Morning meds."

The little white pill didn't look like my omeprazole and it sure as shit wasn't synthetic THC, but I didn't have the ability to ask questions. I picked up the paper cup mechanically because that's what I had seen in the movies, and put it to my lips.

I swallowed my pill without question. I'd find out later it was an antipsychotic.

Without any instruction, I opened my mouth and lifted my tongue to show her that I had swallowed the pill. My room was simple, another raised, rounded plastic rectangle without anything on top of it partnered with a single toilet, no door, and a closet that had no hangers and one shelf. Next to the bed was a shelf to put a cup of water and a blue folder, with my name written in black Sharpie. It felt distinctly like the first day of kindergarten.

Are you excited to make new friends, Katie?

Not really.

To my surprise, I could roam the hall freely. I left the safety of my single cell and walked the long hallway of what would be my home for the next six days. I had not planned on spending my wedding anniversary separated from my husband, but there I was breaking through to the other side, alone and afraid. The halls were lined with various pieces of art: photographs of close-up flowers and birds flying over exotic horizons.

Each room seemed to house one or two patients, but all lacked any sense of privacy. I felt as though I was walking through a fog, and I felt my pulse increasing with a sense of dread: I was suddenly tachycardic.

Tachycardia simply refers to a heartbeat faster than one hundred beats per minute and it felt like a caged bird was trying to escape my chest. My heart was beating faster than normal, and, in hindsight, I know now it was because the antipsychotic stimulated long QT syndrome for me, a heart arrhythmia that can be fatal if untreated. As I roamed that hall, seeking the nurse's station at the very end, I found myself sinking to my knees, the world swimming around me.

"Help," I weakly whispered, fist clenched against my chest.

"Get up. Come on! Up you go!" A nurse appeared from behind the glass, encouraging me to stand.

"I—I can't breathe right." My heart jack hammered away inside my chest.

"Yes, you can. If you can talk, you can breathe." The nurse wasn't listening.

"Get up." Another voice broke through my haze, darker and deeper.

I looked over to my right and saw a balding man, about my age in his mid-thirties, chewing on his nails and shaking his head.

"If you don't get up, they'll shoot you up again. It's just the drugs. Walk it off." He reassured me, not moving.

"That's enough." The nurse admonished my newfound friend.

I took her hand, and stood shakily, getting to the chair next to the strange man. He offered his hand but, before I could take it, the nurse stepped between us with a vitals cart.

"No contact between patients," she chirped as my blood pressure registered 140s/90s and my pulse settled at 125, both of which were unusually high for me.

"You're fine. See – just fine."

"That's not normal for me." I shook my head.

Variations between that conversation happened repeatedly over the next six days. I watched not only as I was dismissed, but as each and every patient was dismissed and diagnosed into boxes that not only didn't fit, but didn't actually help them in any way. During my time in the inpatient unit, I met several characters whom I will never forget, because they reminded me that we are all only a diagnosis away from destruction.

The kind gentleman who spoke up quickly became my tour guide and it seemed that was his role for many of the other patients. He was prone to waxing philosophical and so I internally nicknamed him the Philosopher. The Philosopher spoke with the pressured tones of someone who had a lot on their mind but would lose it if they didn't speak it instantly. It was clear to me his diagnosis was a Bipolar variant, but he seemed saner than half the staff.

"You know what God wants for us?" he asked one day as I was staring out the only window, at the city cemetery below.

"No, what?"

Below us sat an array of patients ranging in age from teenagers to the elderly, eagerly waiting to hear one of the Philosopher's sermons. He was a frequent flier, and he confided in me that he would often "act crazy" because a week inpatient was a vacation compared to the harsh streets or jail cells of the city. Each day he would wax poetic by the window, and he gathered a small following of patients that wanted to listen.

There was The Child, a Hispanic youth with soft eyes and a softer voice, who was prone to panic attacks and desperately craved the attention of his mother. He couldn't have been older than seventeen and he looked to the Philosopher, much like I did, as a guide.

The Mute was not really a mute; he was a sixty-year-old Hispanic man who spoke not a lick of English. I failed to understand how his commitment to an inpatient unit in which no one spoke his language served as anything more than a holding cell, but he did have a knack for the finger-painting.

The Art Critics were a pair of anorexic twenty-something-year-old girls that found friendship within their shared cell. They both were frequent fliers, not just of this facility, but many facilities throughout the country. They were sweet girls, both struggling with self-esteem and stuck in the inpatient unit because neither would eat the daily required meals. You would often find them wandering the lone hall commenting on the art. They said pretending to be a famous art critic not only passed the time, but made them feel important, as if someday their opinions might mean something to someone.

The Karen was a sixty-something-year-old white woman who was serving her third sentence of the year because her paranoia was getting the better of her. She really, really disliked anyone who was "dark," and she was constantly being reprimanded by the nursing staff for causing race issues. On my second-to-last night in the unit, she was supposed to bunk up with a black woman with schizophrenia. The nurses had quite the challenge when she started spitting racial slurs, so I approached the nurse's station and quietly offered to bunk with the black woman. It was the least I could do to spare her from hearing Karen's filth, and I knew that if I appeared helpful, the nursing staff would mark me as well behaved and I would be that much closer to leaving the unit. I will say though, there are few things scarier than closing your eyes and sleeping next to a schizophrenic you only just met twenty minutes ago.

I wondered if she was scared of me, too.

The Rager was a twenty-something-year-old man clearly suffering from anger issues; his exact diagnosis escaped me. He seemed calm enough for long enough, but after only one day on the inside, he started screaming to be freed. The nurses warned him. All the patients reflexively took shelter in their cells. Code Grey was called on him more than anyone that week.

"So, what does God want from us?" The Philosopher asked again.

"To be happy," the Child whispered hopefully, arms tucking his knees close to his chin.

"There is no God," the Rager muttered. No one dared directly contradict him.

"God wants us to be free. He wants us to be naked like children. Like Adam and Eve," the Philosopher pontificated. "He doesn't want us to be bogged down with chemicals or killing each other. He wants us to love each other."

I kept my head down, coloring an owl. My mother had visited me, dropping off a care package with hugs and kisses as if I were just having another summer at fat camp. The cookies she packed were confiscated, and the pajamas she bought me for the remainder of my stay were also kept because they had a drawstring and the phrase, "Drink About It."

We weren't allowed strings in the inpatient facility, and we weren't allowed to talk about drugs or alcohol.

By my third day inpatient, I was withdrawing from my cannabis, and my stomach felt as if it were a blossoming bonfire. While the inpatient crew kept the sedatives coming in the form of Xanax and Zyprexa, somehow my omeprazole was omitted from the regimen. Omeprazole is a proton pump inhibitor that was essential in managing the heartburn and, after about seventy-two hours off of those purple capsules, my stomach became a bubbling acid bath splashing up the backside of my throat and burning my mouth.

I told the nurses I needed the omeprazole. It was never administered.

Going into the fourth day, I woke up a few hours after I fell asleep, chunks of gray meat and cheese erupting from my body from a cheeseburger a nurse forced me to eat under observation. I cried over the toilet bowl; I had warned them I couldn't eat solid food but it was written off as a psychosomatic complaint and not a physical disability. Within seconds, my room lights were turned on and a male attendant appeared in the door frame demanding I stop vomiting.

"Please, I have gastroparesis," I whined pitifully, grease smearing my lips.

"Sure you do, sure you do." He shook his head and ignored my pleas. "Come on, get up now. Do we have a problem here?"

The phrase "do we have a problem" was a code I quickly learned. It meant shape up or we're going to sedate you. I realized I needed to play by their rules if I was ever going to get out of the psych ward. When I was finally admitted into the common area, I looked to the television for guidance, and it blinked to me that I was going to be OK as long as I followed the unwritten rules of the psych ward:

1. Don't get involved in drama. Keep your head down and focus on *you* alone.
2. Take your medicine. Don't argue.
3. Eat your food.

4. Get your exercise by walking.
5. Don't ask questions.
6. Engage in group!

The other patients kept getting in their own ways, and they were no closer to getting discharged out into the real world. I wanted to get out, but I was riddled with paranoia and I was in the right place to be stabilized, I just didn't agree clinically with how they were going about it. According to the hospital staff, we just needed to follow the rules, take our pills, and "be on our best behavior" and if we did that, we'd get privileges.

Privileges were only awarded if you had enough "good behavior points" to be trustworthy. I continued to take my paper cups filled with pills with a thank you and a dutiful opening of the mouth to flaunt my empty oropharynx. What the nursing staff didn't know was that I stopped taking all the pills they offered me on the second day of admission after I experienced that bout of tachycardia.

I wasn't tonguing them; I was slipping them in between the pocket of my front lip and teeth.

I gave them no reason to suspect my disobedience, so each pill was easily hidden away. I knew better than to go to the bathroom immediately after the nurse left. That was an obvious sign of hoarding pills. Instead, I would remain in whatever position I was when I got the drug, coloring or writing, and quietly taking sips of water from my plastic issued vessel.

The vessel was gray and opaque, and no one could ever see inside it.

It was easy to drop the white pills into the water to dissolve over time.

I would ask for regular water refills and no one was the wiser. Similarly, over time, they stopped watching my dinner plates as closely as with that gray cheeseburger. I cut my food into small pieces and ordered soups, mashed potatoes, and toast-based meals to minimize the pain I felt after each forced bite.

Not once did a doctor speak to me while I was inpatient even though I repeatedly asked to speak to a psychiatrist. I didn't meet one until they were discharging me. I really could have used a trauma informed specialist because my memories crystallized during these seven days of insanity. Without my drug regimen for my stomach, I quickly realized my physical symptoms were not the psychosomatic manifestations of childhood sexual assault or complex medical trauma. I was truly physically ill and the more my heartbeat continued to jackhammer and my stomach continued to bubble acid, the more I realized my underlying condition had to be connected to my heart defect.

Vascular, vascular, vascular.

"Get up!" A nurse's voice broke through the din in the common area, this time directed at the Child.

He had fallen to his knees and was hyperventilating.

"I can't," he whimpered.

"Get up right now. Do we have a problem?" The nurse put her hand on her hip; it was almost cartoonish and, even though the first rule of the psych ward floated through my mind, I couldn't not get involved. If she kept escalating, The Child would end up in restraints.

254

"Do we have a problem?" she asked again, towering over him.

"No, we don't." I stood up from my chalk drawing and stood next to him in a few quick strides, "He's fine. Give him a minute."

Before she could chastise me, I dropped down to sit next to him, "Do you want to hold my hand?"

"No contact!" the nurse yelped.

I whipped my head around and the Physician Assistant Kateland spoke confidently, "Do you want to escalate a Code Grey, or do you want me to calm this child down so you don't have to fill out more paperwork today?"

She did a double take and that gave me enough time to focus on him and I asked him, "Hey, what's up?"

"My…My mom. She…she doesn't…she doesn't want…want me," he stuttered, crying as he hid his head in his tucked knees.

One of the Art Critics filled in the rest of the story: he asked for early release but, as he was a minor, his mother needed to sign off on him. She refused, telling him that he was "too much for her to handle at home right now and she needed to think of his little brothers."

He felt abandoned.

He felt alone.

He wasn't wrong.

The nurse let me do my thing because, in just a few short minutes, we went from stuttering to breathing deeply together, to standing up together, to sitting at a table coloring like good boys and girls. No Haldol needed.

"Healer," the Philosopher called me. "That's your name. You're the Healer. You've always been one; I can see it in your past lives."

The Art Critics and the Child nodded in agreement: I listened to them. I made eye contact. I was kind. I was also coming out of the fog of the sedatives, and I realized, as I was freed from all chemical variables, that my pain was real. It was consistent. I knew I would crawl out of this darkness by focusing on my strength: I was a diagnostician.

So what is the diagnosis then?

I had plenty of time to think while I was wasting away in that unit so I decided I would play house; I would play Dr. House, MD. I wrote up a differential board, trying to key into my symptoms and one of the etiologies that had not been explored previously kept popping up in my mind, just like the night I tried to choke back my cherry Tylenol cocktail:

Vascular, vascular, vascular.

We had ruled out autoimmune, infectious, and malignant etiologies but had settled on psychosomatic. I was clearly a crazy woman, and my gastrointestinal symptoms were nothing more than the physical manifestations of a mind gone horribly wrong. Whether that was from the trauma I had uncovered the week before my hospital admission, or whether it was from something else, I simply didn't know.

What I *did* know was that I had a strong suspicion of my underlying diagnosis and I needed to get out of the hospital and onto a computer. I needed to research vascular malformations but, much like the fictional doctor House during the season he was sent to a psych ward, I couldn't do anything until I had broken free from my psychiatric cage. I grew bitter, thinking about how a lifetime of missed diagnoses and the subsequent pain they inflicted would cause anyone to go mad.

I was in the madhouse, and I was really fucking mad.

While we didn't have access to psychiatrists on the inpatient unit, we did have access to art therapists. Once again, I connected with color as a way to calm my nerves. I knew I was getting out of the hospital the day I created a chalk portrait of myself. The counselor encouraged us to create a picture of how we were feeling at that very moment, and I couldn't help but snort to myself. If I really shared how I was feeling, I would never get out of this hospital.

I was pissed off that I fell through the cracks time and again.

I was furious I was in a holding tank of sedatives and fingerpaint.

I was paranoid my life was over, and now that I went nuts, I'd never be considered a respectable clinician again.

When the art therapist asked us to paint ourselves, I painted myself in a lotus position, sitting atop my kayak, with a sun setting behind me. The green spirals that curled from my head, heart, and pelvis contrasted with the choppy waves and diagonal beams of the setting sun. When the counselor asked me what it meant, I smiled dully and obediently:

"This represents me overcoming past traumas by integrating the tools I've learned here and through my spiritual practices over the years to move into the future, which is represented by the sun over choppy water."

He beamed.

I beamed back, mimicking him, mirroring his body language and his verbal language just like I learned in the Applied Behavioral Analysis group so many years ago; conform or perish.

The day I was released from the hospital, my mind was still cracked, and my vascular system was still broken, but I had been baptized in the fires of insanity and I was aware for the first time in my life. I was still very fragile, but I knew I needed to push forward past the trauma and start a vascular evaluation.

I had come this far; I wasn't going to give up now.

Kate's Anatomy

"I'd like you to order an abdominal ultrasound with duplex, please." I couldn't make eye contact with the doctor, but I needed her to order this test.

"Why?" the doctor wondered idly, "What are you thinking?"

"MALS. Median Arcuate Ligament Syndrome. Dunbar Syndrome. My symptoms match the triad perfectly and the test is an easy outpatient procedure."

Described as a triad of unintentional weight loss, nausea with vomiting, and epigastric abdominal pain (pain above the stomach), MALS refers to a syndrome in which the Median Arcuate Ligament (MAL) compresses the aorta. The MAL is a fibrous muscular band of the diaphragm at the level of the thoracic/lumbar junction of the spine. Everyone has a MAL but not everyone develops MALS.

There are a few different theories floating around as to why some people develop symptoms including congenital (being born that way) or it can be acquired after abdominal trauma. Examples of trauma to the abdomen include surgical scarring or blunt trauma. When the celiac artery is compressed over time, the celiac ganglion (nerve bundle) gets irritated, enlarged, scarred, and eventually dies resulting in paralysis of the stomach (gastroparesis is a symptom, not a diagnosis).

I felt like I was presenting a case to my attending, and I was instantly transported back to graduate school. I didn't like the feeling and it was compounded because the stakes were mine to lose. I feared this doctor lumped me into one of the categories of hypochondriac patients, women who had been sexually assaulted and now were prone to all types of psychosomatic complaints. The only thing I had to stand on was my medical degree, and it felt to me as if my credibility were waning by the day after my nervous breakdown, despite my previous volunteering with the Health Department.

"That's an incredibly rare diagnosis." She was skeptical.

Rarely diagnosed does not mean rare, but I wasn't in a position to argue semantics with her. I wanted this workup; I needed this workup. She advised me that even if my vascular ultrasound were positive, there is no cure for MALS.

The first clinical references to MALS were documented in 1917 by Benjamin Lipshultz, M.D., who wrote a composite study on the anatomical variations of the celiac artery seen during dissections. Little was done with this finding until the 1960s when Dr. PT Harjola described a syndrome of compression of the celiac artery that presented with nausea, vomiting, and abdominal pain. The vague condition finally got a namesake in 1965 when Dr. J. David Dunbar reported a successful surgical repair of the compressed celiac artery, resulting in improved symptoms for fifteen of his patients.

Not only was my doctor uninformed regarding this rare disease, but she was also giving me information that was outdated by nearly 100 years. If I was right about my condition, I did have treatment options that could be successful. I was adamant though and for the first time in my life I advocated for myself without wavering because I was bolstered by knowledge she didn't have. I was bolstered by other patients' testimonies.

After my discharge from the psych unit, I returned to my youthful medical approaches of scouring medical media and the library while actively searching for gainful employment. I needed health insurance if I wanted to confirm my suspicions. While the books held little more than passing sentences referencing Dunbar Syndrome, it was in social media and primetime television that I found my answer.

Online, as The Write Assistant, I connected with patients from all around the globe with similar symptoms. I made so many friends online. One of these friends sent me a link to watch "Everyday Angel," an episode from Grey's Anatomy. This episode aired in the fifteenth season and featured a patient who was plagued with the same symptoms as I. This fictional patient developed food-related anxiety and, after batteries of tests come up negative, she is left desperate and bitter, biting at the medical team that offers her care when Dr. Grey is not available in the episode.

I snorted, of course our fictional heroes aren't available! It's not often we get to meet our heroes, and it looked like this character was also out of luck.

Dr. Bailey, the doctor who ultimately cracked this fictional-ized patient case, informed the angry patient, while she might not be the magical Dr. Grey, she is the attending who taught her, so she best mind her manners if they were going to work together to figure out her clinical curiosities. If only I had a team of female doctors with that type of tenacity! In the real world, the one choked by insurance policies run by people who have never prac-ticed medicine a day in their lives, you don't get that kind of care.

After I finished the episode, bawling my eyes out, I googled the condition's name, Median Arcuate Ligament Syndrome and a flood of information opened up to me in social media sub-groups.

Did you know that those prime-time dramas are sometimes based on real people?

The woman who inspired this episode was not only still alive, but she was active in the social media groups. We connected. She shared that years ago she had traveled for a vascular surgeon who was willing to surgically repair these cases. She shared with me that she was one of his first MALS success stories in the United States and she had been eating regular food for the past several years. She told me I shouldn't give up hope.

I soaked up all the knowledge I could from her and from the support groups she sent my way.

I just needed confirmation.

I just needed this one ultrasound to tell me whether or not my celiac artery was kinked.

If it was kinked, just like a garden hose, the liquid wouldn't get where it needed to go. The celiac artery supplies the stomach, liver, pancreas, and parts of the intestines, and, if compressed over time, would cause severe pain, weight loss, and failure to thrive. While controversial, it was recognized as a congenital vascular malformation that occurred in up to a third of known autopsies, but was only considered to be symptomatic in less than 1% of the population.

If you were part of that 1%, though, the pain was likened to end-stage pancreatic cancer. You were constantly experiencing asphyxiation of your gastrointestinal tract, and I realized that I had been living with that type of pain, intermittently, throughout my whole life. Severe exacerbations in symptoms would often be triggered by a blunt trauma to the abdomen and, after I finished watching her episode, tears in my eyes, I remembered flying through the air that Thanksgiving week when my steering column failed.

The gastroenterologist relented and with a sigh, agreed to order the duplex ultrasound. She cautioned me again, if it were positive she wouldn't treat that condition but she would refer me out to vascular. I thanked her and left that office proud because I spoke up and got a doctor to listen long enough to order the test I needed.

A few weeks later, I sat naked from the waist up waiting for an ultrasound technician to confirm my suspicion. Before I lied down, though, I took my cell phone out and snapped a picture. It felt like something to remember.

As the gel chilled my belly, the technician apologized and made small talk. She grew quiet as she moved the wand across my belly and told me to hold as deep a breath as I could. Her eyebrows wrinkled and I asked her what she saw.

"You'll need to talk to the doctor about the results." She gave me a standard response.

"I understand." I nodded, but then I started sharing my story with her. "You're a doctor?" She arched an eyebrow.

"Physician Assistant, actually. I practice with the Health Department now, just a few towns over." I bluffed my way with some overblown clout. "My GI doesn't believe in MALS and, frankly, I just needed to find someone to order the test. I'm the one who figured out the differential and I'm betting my life that I'm right."

"OK, so you're a provider." She looked around, "So between you and me, this is the worst case of MALS I've ever seen. See this hook shape here?"

She pointed to a very dramatic U on my ultrasound. "Take a deep breath in."

As I did, the U constricted even more dramatically and I exhaled, watching the hose unkink and the blood flow through. We did it again. And again. The blood flow was cut in half. Every single time I took a deep breath, I was choking myself: I was right.

I thanked her for her professional courtesy and she left me in the room alone to get dressed. When she came back to discharge me, she found me in a puddle of tears at the table. They were tears of joy tinged with bittersweet fear of what came next. Now that I confirmed my diagnosis, I was ready to face my real prognosis. Once I composed myself, I admitted that I had been recently hospitalized for a nervous breakdown.

She shook her head knowingly, and advised me, "I can't tell you how many women I see in here that finally get their pain validated. You were never crazy."

Racing home, I went back to my emails to see which doctor my new online friend recommended. Shockwaves coursed over me as I realized the doctor she loved and swore by was none other than a vascular surgeon in my backyard. He was only twenty minutes from my house.

Was this the physician priest I had been praying for all along?

As Long as the Baby Is Healthy

"As long as the baby is healthy, nothing else matters."

My shoulders stiffen, my brow creases, and I inhale sharply every time I hear some variation of this phrase. Health is important, but when we focus the entire worth of someone's experience on how healthy they are, we are implicitly demeaning the inherent value of those with less health.

Now I know what you are thinking, "That's not what I meant! It's normal to wish for a healthy baby. What's wrong with you?"

"Normal" has never been the friend of the medically disadvantaged.

We need to stop equating health with blessings in general conversation.

When you are living with a chronic illness, you're often already on the outside. You feel lonely when you can't participate, for whatever reason, and it accumulates starting in childhood. However, it is the unnecessary reinforcement of health as the penultimate perpetuated by adults around you that starts the "sick is less" snowball. Never had this realization hit me so squarely in the gut than when I was practicing medicine, waiting to be seen by this magical MALS surgeon, whom I thought held the key to my salvation.

Diagnosis finally in hand, I was spurred to return to medicine for health insurance. I left my volunteer position at the Health Department, trading it for a paying job at a for profit retail urgent care clinic. I was practicing medicine in the same city as my potential physician priest and this guaranteed he was in network.

The urgent care was desperate for clinicians as the COVID19 pandemic continued to rage on and they were happy to take me on, even though I was still struggling physically. They didn't ask too many questions about my past and looked the other way when I tested positive for THC on the pre-employment drug screen. I hid my symptoms the best I could by drinking Boost protein shakes and keeping Zofran in my pocket for when the waves of nausea would hit me and if I were too sick to present to a shift, I had less qualms calling out now.

"As long as the baby is healthy, nothing else matters."

Every time I hear that phrase, I will gently clear my throat and represent the invisible ill. It is my perilous hope the room will remember, at least for a moment, that, despite all the well wishes, sometimes those wishes wither on the vine, and you're left with a miracle that grows up to be a mirage.

As my workup with the vascular surgeon loomed large in my mind's eye, I kept thinking about all the cases swirling around me and the language we used to talk about our patients. This was brought to a head, for me, when a family friend experienced dismissal at the hands of her pediatrician as a first-time momma.

Her 15-month-old son was diagnosed with Type I diabetes but was initially dismissed by the pediatric team. The young boy developed diabetic ketoacidosis, a potentially deadly state in which the blood sugar is too high and ketones spill into the urine, requiring emergency stabilization with IV fluids and insulin.

He was healthy. Then he wasn't.

Just like me.

Now what?

"As long as the baby is healthy, nothing else matters."

Now we introduce needles and numbers, dosages and directions, restrictions and remedies…Now we introduce inspirational hero worship and remove any sense of personal privacy as you and your family are in the "less than" space.

But, if you hope, wish, pray, swallow, or inject long enough, you'll get back to that place where nothing else matters.

The place where everything is bright and clear.

The bright place where family and friends smile with delight when you walk up unhindered, rather than the dark place you are now, where the light behind others' eyes has dimmed and been replaced with something much more saccharin. Something sentimentally bitter and sweet because they only wish you well, after all.

It happens every day, in every clinic, in every state around this country, but cases like this still bring me back to my own childhood. And now that I was waiting for the definitive consultation after thirty-five years, I just kept reliving those childhood fears. These casual dismissals remind me that once upon a time, I was a sick kid on a cold table, wondering what I could do to make them stop bringing me into those offices and operating theaters.

What could I do to get back to that place of "healthy" the adults were always talking about?

What could I do to get away from the place I was, the dark place where "nothing else matters"?

I can speak up, now that I was trained up and on the other side of my nervous breakdown. So I started speaking up more. I was using my white coat to coach others online that their words mattered and, for the first time in my life, I was focused on myself and insisting I get the care I would offer others. I counted down the days to my consultation, praying I wouldn't be dismissed again, I meditated on that phrase that seemed to haunt my family friends.

"As long as the baby is healthy…"

This is a well-wish we could have always done without, during my childhood and so many others, so let me propose an alternative blessing to bestow:

"As long as we love each other, then nothing else matters."

I Spit

"I spit."

The words came out of the tiny tot's trembling mouth with surprising clarity, and I had only a fracture of a second to ask, "What?" before he angled his head back and promptly spit at me.

Oh, no, no, little man. You did NOT just spit at me.

When working in urgent care, you often meet people at their worst. Generally speaking, humans do not act their best when faced with discomfort. The fear that can be conjured in a medical office is significant, so it's not surprising that a five-year-old with a chin laceration was not the pinnacle of politeness.

His mother brought him in just before eight in the evening, noting he fell off the bed and cracked his chin. He had an abundance of energy, shared mom, and he was a bit of a handful. She really didn't know where he got the energy, because he certainly didn't listen to her when she told him to calm down for bedtime. She leaned in and admitted conspiratorially that he never really listened to her and it was just frankly easier to let him do what he wanted when he wanted. She shrugged, and I sighed.

I took a closer look. The bleeding had stopped long before they arrived at my clinic, but it was a nice little laceration that could have been closed with a stitch. Theoretically, it could have been closed with a stitch. That is until my patient started engaging in biological warfare with spit missiles.

I turned to the mother, from the furthest point in the room, and said, "I don't play that game. I'm going to step out and give you a few moments with him."

I was still counting down the days to my Celiac Block, an interventional radiology procedure to confirm if I was a candidate for MALS surgery, and I was not in the mood to risk spit missiles. Until I completed the Celiac Block, I couldn't risk even a minor illness delaying my workup, and I was fairly fearful of the swirling COVID-19 and influenza infections in the community.

As I stood outside the room waiting for mom to calm her kiddo down, a scary thought hit me:

What if the surgeon gets sick? What if he dies from COVID-19 before the surgery is scheduled?

I pushed the intrusive thought from my mind, and braced myself to return to the kid with expert aim. I expected the mother to give him a little pep talk, a hug, and maybe hold his hand. He had no outstanding medical or sensory needs, and it was clear he was a very intelligent child; he was just scared. He did not want me touching his wound, and he was simply trying to defend himself. Now, it is clear to me in retrospect: this is where the visit went horribly, horribly wrong.

Children are never at fault for their behavior.

I'm going to repeat that line: Children are never at fault for their behavior.

As much as I was worked up at the idea of a kiddo spitting at me, I understood logically that he was only doing the best he could with what he had at that time. Parents need to set good examples of experiencing discomfort so that their children realize that, while they are uncomfortable, they are not in danger when in a medical space. Fear tactics have no place in pediatric medicine. One of my biggest pet peeves as a clinician is when parents use me (or my staff) as a threat: "Behave or you'll get a shot!"

Frankly, with that type of framing, I'd spit, too.

I took a deep breath in, steeled myself with a package of surgical glue and steri-strips, and prepared for round two. I opened the door to find him pinned against the table by his mother's right hand. Her magnificently manicured neon orange acrylics framed his face with a crab-like spindling.

He proceeded to spit through his mother's fingers.

"Do it," Mom said. "Do it now while I've got him pinned!"

"Do what?" I looked horrified at the scene. "Please let your child up."

"But he'll start spitting at you if I do," she warned before letting her hand up, and true to her warning, he did start spitting at me.

"I SPIT!"

To detail the remainder of the meltdown would be excessive, but, needless to say, I used the age-old trick clinicians have been using on wary children for years: sugar.

It was actually the patient's sister who spoke up first, identifying the potential for a candy at the end of the visit. She was a seven-year-old who was over the visit before it began, and she kept telling her brother to knock it off so she could get candy. I told her that she could have candy at the end of the visit.

"Can I have candy?" His voice peeped out again, spittle spilling from the corner of his suddenly smiling visage.

"No, no you cannot. Because you spit at me."

The mother looked at me in disbelief. The children looked at me in disbelief. I froze in fear as I realized I just got petty with a pediatric patient.

"You can have candy after I put a Band-Aid on the boo-boo," I offered, backpedaling just a bit. I am only human, after all, and I'm only a human who barely avoided a spit bath three times.

He side-eyed me. I side-eyed him.

He let me come closer, the idea of candy dangling between us as a protective shield. Within a few minutes the wound was covered with surgical glue, a few steri-strips, and a Band-Aid with an appropriate cartoon character. I was exhausted but I wasn't contaminated.

"Where's my candy?" Both children growled when I returned to the room with discharge papers. In the few minutes I'd been gone, they destroyed the room further as they climbed the walls in anticipation of their escape into the night.

"Here, you each get two lollipops! One for each hand!" I smiled.

As I watched them leave, patched up and perked up with the age-old medicine of candy, I shook my frustration and disgust off with a few deep breaths. Medicine can be traumatic, for everyone involved, but it doesn't have to be. Parents influence how their child perceives the world and by using positive framing tech-niques, in and out of the clinic, we can minimize unnecessary stress and anxiety.

At the end of the day, even though the little one was a spitter, he was still just a child and didn't deserve to be pinned by his mother or denied candy.

No, in cases like this, children always get candy.

Idly, I wondered if the vascular surgeon's office had lollipops.

Celiac Block Rock

The date was set for my Celiac Block.

I needed to be at the hospital by 7 AM that morning, nothing to eat or drink for the twelve hours prior (no problem!), but my husband could *not* come in due to COVID-19 restrictions. The fact that I'd be facing this workup mostly alone hadn't really hit me until the night before the procedure.

I was distraught.

I didn't think I could do it, but I had no other choice.

The only way out is through…

I reached out to my current primary care provider, a woman who was little more than a placeholder and had no real interest in my case, and she dutifully faxed over a controlled substance meant to sedate: my old friend Xanax. She never even asked me about my psychiatric history. She had no idea I tried to kill myself previously with cherry flavored Xanax and, frankly, I didn't offer that information to her.

I was already shaking just thinking about the needles going into my spine as the procedure includes two injections of a steroid and an anesthetic directly into my mid-back. Basically, if the injection alleviated my symptoms and allowed me to eat food without pain, I would be a candidate for surgical repair.

When we pulled into the pharmacy and saw the drive through was closed, I told my husband I'd just pop in and get it myself because I just needed to move. The excess energy was radiating off of me and I was sure I was giving off signs of madwoman. My eyes were still red from crying earlier.

I walked down the brightly lit center aisle of the pharmacy, but, to my surprise, an elderly woman kept purposefully walking toward me, keeping intense eye contact. Her wide blue eyes were framed by the same style of glasses my Oma used to wear, her curled white hair cushioned gently by a silk scarf of similar style. The resemblance was uncanny, and I didn't want anyone, never mind a specter from my past, to see me in this state. I looked down and tried to avoid her, but she stopped immediately in front of me and wouldn't let me pass her.

"Um, excuse me?" I tried to step out of her way.

"You're going to be OK."

I did a double-take and, as I looked into her pale, watery blue eyes, she said in her trembling voice, "Everything is going to be OK."

"I…I don't." I shook my head, moving backward, but she followed me, her steps mirroring mine.

I felt my resolve crumbling in the confusion. The two of us stood, suspended in the middle of the pharmacy, staring at each other. And the longer I looked at her curled hair under the silk wrap, the more confused I became. She kept her gaze steady on mine, smiling gently, and it seemed that, beyond those wire-framed glasses, her eyes were enlarging into pools of water and beckoning me to swim into them.

I didn't say it out loud, but someone whispered inside me, *"Is that you, Oma?"*

She smiled, nodded once, and walked away, not uttering another word.

I almost dropped to my knees in the aisle and prayed right there.

I choked back a sob and hid my pink eyes brimming with tears under my black sunglasses, even though it was nighttime. It was a sign; it had to be. I wasn't looking for them, not really, but they kept popping up in ways I just couldn't ignore. The encounter left me shaken, but, after the initial shock wore off, I felt a sense of peace come over me. I told my husband immediately, but his atheist mind wouldn't entertain the idea of a ghost in CVS. When I told my mother, she believed me and reminded me that my Oma would tell me, "The only way out was through."

I was comforted by the thought my ancestors decided to pop up to wish me well once before my procedure. At least, that's the story I told myself that night to help fall asleep. I also said a silent prayer to Hypnos, god of dreams and anesthesia, as I slipped his holy wafer of benzodiazepine beneath my trembling tongue.

The next morning arrived and it was a frozen winter day. We arrived at the hospital entrance and my husband dropped me off. I prepared myself to face the building, tears gathering at the edges of my eyes not just from the anxiety, but from the sheer bitterness of the windchill. My husband remained in our car for the entirety of my procedure, and my thoughts flashed to him, imagining how cold he would be waiting outside; it's not like he could keep the car running for the three hours I was expected to be inside. I moved my way through the registration line until finally the receptionist asked me to take off my mask for a stone-faced photo identification.

The bulb flashed and I disassociated.

The next thing I remember is urinating in a cup, providing a pregnancy sample before they would place the IV line. I laughed ironically; I still couldn't have sex. I could barely breathe without collapsing into a pile of tears. The pregnancy test was predictably negative.

I will be forever grateful to the team that conducted my celiac block. They answered my prayers to Hypnos. They were patient and kind and listened to my story. They offered anecdotes of others who came through those hallowed halls and went on to successfully survive the MALS reconstruction surgery.

I felt a tinge of hope as the twist of the IV went deeper, saline flowing to establish the line.

To distract myself, I took a selfie and posted it to my social media channels along with the lyrics I was binging on repeat. The Write Assistant channel kept growing and I was encouraged by my fellow rare disease friends online. One of my favorite singers crooned in my earbuds as I laid back, crying silently as I begged for the numbness to hit me.

I looked down at the saline plug in my hand; the IV was placed in my right hand, and not the crook of my elbow as I'd hoped as those tend to be less painful. I started to panic a little as the anesthesiologist came in, introducing himself as the doctor that would be conducting the procedure. He was a slight, slender white male with wire-framed glasses and a mildly gingered appearance.

He smiled warmly and reassured me the best he could.

He went over the basics of the procedure one more time. I was going to be wheeled into the interventional radiology suite because we were going to inject a large needle into the base of my celiac nerve plexus in the thoracic spine. That needle was going to contain a small portion of a numbing agent, lidocaine, and a steroid, prednisone, that was theoretically going to paralyze the affected nerve bundle.

You see, over time, as the median arcuate ligament restricts the celiac artery, vein, and nerve bundle, the nerves grow bigger and angrier. The restriction causes further loss of blood flow resulting in necrotic tissue if left untreated for long time periods. While the Celiac Block wouldn't treat my symptoms, it would block them by rendering my brain physically incapable of reading the chemical signals of distress my gastrointestinal system was generating. The hope was that, after I was wheeled out of the interventional radiology suite, I'd be struck with hunger and the magical ability to eat all the foods again.

I was placed face down on a gurney, both arms strapped above my head, cramping my shoulders slightly. The pressure on my abdomen was overwhelming, and I started to hyperventilate, wondering how the hell I'd stay still and why the ever-loving fuck I wasn't more sedated.

What was in those IV lines?

Whatever it was, it wasn't affecting me, and the anesthesiologist told me to do my very best to stay very, very still. While others describe a sedated experience, I remained stone-cold sober for the entirety of my procedure.

I felt the cold swab of iodine and the room suddenly smelled brown.

The way I experience the world is sometimes hard to convey, but words and places can be associated with colors and smells. For me, normally, hospitals smell and look yellow. The yellow edges of my periphery darkened as the cold press of the cleansing agent was replaced by the tight initial sensation of a pinprick. The pinprick quickly expanded into an unbelievably deep sensation of penetration.

"Hold your breath," the surgeon stated.

"Ah!" I whimpered, holding my breath on the inhale, closing my eyes tightly and chanting lyrics inside my head.

...*Drink back the numb, drink back the numb, drink back the numb, drink back the numb...*

There was a whir as the machine holding me up moved underneath the CT scan so the surgeon could confirm his needle was exactly where it needed to be. It was.

"A little pinch now," the surgeon continued.

"AH!" I screamed as the needle flooded the right side of my spine with burning.

My eyes flashed white behind closed lids, and I felt a wave of nausea hit the back of my throat: nothing but putrid air pushing up against my lips. There was nothing inside me to give up anymore.

"That's it, halfway done on this side." He spoke again but I barely registered his syllables.

The burning continued, and it felt like the right side of my body was cramping into a ball while simultaneously expanding into hot white light. Was this supposed to feel this way? Was this my imagination? Was I being dramatic?

"All done on this side. Take a few deep breaths; we're going to prep the other side." He gave me a reprieve.

Some part of me appreciated the verbal narrative even though I couldn't vocalize. I shifted slightly under the heavy weight of my medicated body, and I opened my eyes to peek around the room. That was a mistake. To my left was a surgical tray, the blue sterile cloth topped with a variety of instruments.

I gagged on grotesque yellow brown air again, and a nurse patted the hand that wasn't stuck like a bloody pincushion. The room turned a darker shade of brown and I felt the iodine wash over my back and my mind for the second time. I practiced my deep breathing, the steady flow learned in too many yoga classes to count, but soon the doctor warned me it was time to hold it once again.

A second prick and the left side of my spine was on fire.

I was violently nauseous, and the cramps exploded to include both sides of my body. There was nowhere for me to escape this new pain. This new, green-brown, violent churning in my abdomen radiated into the back of my pelvis and I was instantly exhausted even though it was barely nine in the morning. I was limp as they wheeled me out of the radiology suite and into my private room.

Someone handed me a menu and said, "Order."

I laughed as I retched bile into the blue emesis bag I kept in my lap, wondering how they could even suggest such a thing. Tears filled my eyes, and I debated if I made a mistake. I couldn't even consider food; my stomach was filled with a new feeling, and it wasn't good. It was disgusting. It was worse than before.

The nurses encouraged me to order anyway, and I asked them if I could wait just a few minutes and start by sipping on some water. One of the more interesting clinical symptoms of MALS is that drinking water causes severe pain. I hadn't had a plain glass of water in years and so sipping on it, it was a delicacy. I started with clear sips as I waited on my hospital cafeteria tray to be delivered.

I texted my husband, "I don't think it worked."

Later, he told me how his heart sank as he sat outside in the car, turning the heater on every twenty minutes or so to stay warm, waiting for the news.

But, *ye of little faith...*

The nurses waited, checking in on me and my vitals every fifteen minutes. The second half of this procedure was eating and comparing my pain pre and post block. If I didn't eat at all, the entire thing would be in vain. The food tray came up to my room and, to my surprise, I started to cut the food into little pieces, and those little pieces started to make their way into my mouth.

Then down my esophagus.

Then into my stomach.

I realized my stomach wasn't immediately regurgitating. Sure, I was nauseous and crampy, but I just had two giant needles jammed into the middle of my spine…and I was eating!

On that cold January morning, after years of nothing more than nibbles, I successfully ate the following meal:

1 Chicken Caesar Salad + Newman's Salad Dressing
1/2 Orange
1 Strawberry
3 Pineapple Spears
3 Honeydew Slices
3 Cantaloupe Slices
1 Red Grape

All it took was the right diagnosis.

The nurses and anesthesiologist cheered me on as they disconnected the IV line. They knew the next step was my afternoon consultation with the esteemed physician priest, the vascular surgeon, so they wished me luck and I wished them safety. I nearly bounced into the car eager to tell my husband my text was wrong! It worked! It really worked!

"I ate food!"

We listened to my Celiac Block Rock playlist on repeat, but, this time, I was chomping joyfully on a Brown Asian Pear as we drove to the surgeon's office.

I was ecstatic.

Two hours later, I was sitting in the surgeon's office, waiting nervously for him to enter.

Would he agree the block was a success?

There's a well-known stereotype that surgeons don't have the best bedside manner; they lack the bells and whistles and gentle touch of pediatricians, for example. This surgeon was no different.

This vascular surgeon was a quiet, reserved man who was focused on the pathology more so than the patient and in a lot of ways that's exactly the kind of person you'd want for a surgery. In each of my interactions with him, I found myself at odds with his bedside manner because it differed so much from my own, but I also wanted someone who was confident in treating this condition. He was logical and all about the facts, so again, exactly the kind of man you'd want cutting you open.

He pushed on my belly, at the epigastric center and asked, "Pain?"

"No! Not really, no." I beamed at him, and while there was some nausea lingering, the ball of pressure that normally sat on my chest and upper abdomen was thankfully gone, gone, gone!

"You have the anatomy for MALS. You have the symptoms and you are responsive to the block. You are a candidate for surgery. If you want to schedule it, my office manager can take it from here. Do you have any questions for me before I send her in?"

His voice was clipped and flat, and I could tell he'd given this script many, many times before.

I nodded, showing understanding but at the same time, I was flabbergasted by how nonchalantly he confirmed my diagnosis.

Didn't he understand it took me a lifetime to get here?

"Yes. Yes. I want to get on the waitlist." I nodded emphatically, tears of joy sparkling in my eyes.

He sent his office manager in to replace him; he had other much more important things to do. I would find over the course of my time getting to know this doctor that his bedside manner left me feeling alone most of the time. The office manager was a blonde woman with a bright smile and I found she always wore the best dresses. She carried that office in a wonderful way because she offered kindness, a willingness to listen, and allowed me to reminisce about food. She provided the gentle touch and bedside manner I was craving, and I was grateful for her influence during my evaluation.

As I left the office, she told me to start planning menus again with my husband with a smile.

This was quickly followed up with a cautionary warning though, not to get my hopes too high. There was a long waitlist. The wait was quoted at close to six months but when I got the call for surgery, I would need to go. It was a bit like transplant medicine and if you hesitated, your spot would be given to the next in line.

I told her I understood, and I was absolutely ready.

That night, my husband and I ordered from the Greek restaurant I had been eying since we'd moved back into town. I had pork souvlaki and while it didn't sit very well with me, I had it, and that was a triumph! I also had baklava, and gyro meat drizzled with tzatziki sauce, cucumbers, and tomatoes on a pillowy soft pita.

I was saved.

I was saved for ten days, but by the eleventh day I woke up at 5:30 AM with that familiar rumble of pain in my epigastric center. It was the hollow lava that needed to erupt, and I knew with unshakable certainty: I had always had MALS, and this was the only way forward.

My husband and I sat down and made a budget for the next six months. I could pick up an extra shift per week and we could pocket the money. We'd apply for short-term disability and family medical leave because in six months, I'd have been with the urgent care company for a year and my benefits would be in full swing.

We'd be OK.

We just had to make it for six more months.

I continued to build my urgent care practice, and I found my confidence had returned, and grew stronger than before. I had cracked my case! I just needed to make it to July and then I'd finally have my medical independence.

I was at the urgent care clinic working when I got the call for my surgery. I was training a new provider. I missed the actual call, so when the email popped up in my inbox with the date and confirmation request, I was in the middle of explaining how to code a nursing visit to our newest clinician.

"Sorry, let me just check this." I opened the email but felt hot because she was reading over my shoulder. I felt lightheaded as the words in front of me swirled from black to gray to white.

"I…I…I…" I stuttered incoherently.

My new colleague looked at me confused, "Everything OK?"

"That says…that…that…" I took a deep breath and composed myself, "That says…March 16th, right?"

Her eyes followed my fingers to the pixelated date I was pointing to, and she nodded. "Yeah, why?"

"That's…that's…six weeks. Not six months."

The Resurrectionist

Somewhere suspended within this muscle memory matrix of
manifest destiny,
My DNA decided to go rogue.
A kink in the system set me up for a story from which there is
no escape,
Because the plot has always been pointed,
And as sharp as original sin.

– Kateland Kelly, hospital journal excerpt

In the 1800s, grave robbers used to steal corpses for anatomists to study so they could understand the human body better. These men, and sometimes women, would sneak off to tombs after dark to resurrect bodies into teaching tools for medical schools. They were given the moniker of Resurrectionists. MALS, even if acknowledged by the medical establishment, is only considered to be symptomatic in 1% of the cases. Patients are often told pursuing a diagnosis isn't worthwhile, just like I was, because many doctors just don't believe in the anatomy.

They don't believe that this type of vascular malformation is capable of causing such pain.

I can't help but wonder if the people who once studied bodies looked closer, and if they listened to the stories of the wailing women, and men, then maybe we wouldn't be exploring this brave new world of medicine in the 2020s. Dr. Lipshultz listened. Dr. Harjola listened. So did Dr. Dunbar. Maybe we would have spared generations of monsters, Frankenstein's monsters, if only the rest of the medical community had looked at the anatomy properly and listened to our collectively lived experiences.

I was afraid of surgery and I was afraid of dying. I was preparing myself for the distinct possibility that I wouldn't be coming out of the hospital and, even though my husband tried to kiss away my fears, he didn't understand the dangers of living inpatient the way I did. I joked with my best friend that I was like Jesus, going to sleep for a few days and then coming back when the going was good. I was jesting out of desperation.

I was really thinking of Bobby, my pediatric cancer patient, dying in their hospital bed so many years prior and I was ramping up my dark humor to cope. The only way out was through, though. So, with a heavy heart, I kissed my husband goodbye one more time and walked into the hospital with a nurse at my side and my ancestors behind me. What happened next is a bit of a blur.

While the average length of stay for a Celiac Ganglionectomy was quoted at somewhere between five and seven days, I spent more than three times that length hospitalized with complications: twenty-two days to be exact.

The morning of the surgery, I was terrified. My vascular surgeon did little to calm my fears, as he was only focused on getting consent. His green mask tented as he spoke, "Are you certain you are ready to proceed with surgery today?"

He was impeccable at getting informed consent. I consented. Sometimes it felt like he was trying to convince me not to do it because, as any good surgeon knows, selecting your caseload is key to positive success rates. He didn't want to add a failure to his tally, and I didn't want to be such a failure so if I had any hesitation, he warned, I shouldn't proceed.

"Yes, I'm ready." I nodded. "The only thing to do is jump over the moon."

He wasn't one to wax poetic over my insertion of *Rent* lyrics, so he moved on to the surgical suite to leave the nursing staff to prepare me. They wheeled me into the operating theater and an anesthesiologist towered above me as I laid on the gurney. He took my left arm and strapped it down; I was halfway crucified, and I felt the nostalgic stab of stigmata in my wrists. An echo of childhood...

"What are you doing?" I protested as he prepared to strap my other arm into medical bondage.

"Just getting ready to put you under." He was quick in his actions and curt in his tones. All business here.

If you've never had general anesthesia, it's hard to describe the dissociation that comes from being awake and present in one room, to not. He lowered a green mask to my face, drugs hissing from the hose, and as I inhaled the yellow scented medication the room swirled and I was gone, gone, gone...

Beep...beep...beep...beep...

...hours later I was resurrected with a new anatomy.

Through the haze of anesthesia, I returned to the land of the living, split open with an abdominal incision that started just below the center of my rib cage and ended just above my belly button. My eyes failed to focus at first, and I felt a dull thrum of my heartbeat synced in tune to the cacophony of bells and whistles monitoring me. I looked to my left and a sink held gloves and tools. Behind me, a collection of IV fluids dripped into my left hand, impaled by a butterfly access.

I blinked back tears; the color yellow flooded my senses. It was an overwhelming sensation that flitted behind my weak eyelids but permeated the scene when I opened them. The world was yellow, and I was a half-baked egg, quivering in my vulnerability. This is the only way I know how to describe the feeling of dipping my toes back into the world after I so intimately tasted oblivion once more. My husband squeezed my hand on my right, and after he reassured me I made it out and was in recovery. I fell back asleep, lullabied by the beeping and booping of machines and too drugged by Dilaudid to care about anything.

...beep...beeep...beeeeeep...

When I awoke next, I felt what could only be described as a hornet burrowing into my left hand, the back of my palm stinging with the fire of Hymenoptera. I tried shaking my arm, desperate to fling the yellow monster off of me, but as my filmy eyes opened fully, I saw no insect on my extremity and realized it was a misinterpretation of my physical surroundings. The back of my left

291

wrist was connected to my narcotic pain management pump and it stung like a mother.

Before I went into that hospital, I was relatively narcotic naive, but inpatient was an entirely different story. I was given a direct line to as many opioids as I could handle with a handy-dandy push button for when I needed another hit through an intravenous narcotic pump. I could get a hit of Dilaudid every six minutes.

The sedative and constipatory side effects of mainlining that many narcotics in a post-op period meant that I was supposed to start walking ASAP, and I needed to get my fiber otherwise I was at risk for bowel obstructions. Looking down at my abdomen, my pale bloated eggshell belly beneath the blue smock, I gasped when I saw little silhouettes of ruby red blossom through. My surgical site was leaking, and my left hand was still stinging with the imaginary insect.

I desperately hit the nurse call button, an action I would repeat ad nauseum over the next ten days at this hospital, only resulting in pissing off their nursing staff.

"Ice, please." I begged and looked down at my belly when a nurse finally entered the room, "Something is wrong."

She didn't introduce herself but she looked at the IV and said it looked fine to her. I whimpered and told her it didn't feel right. She didn't say much else after that but, according to my husband, she didn't return with that ice for nearly forty minutes.

As the imaginary hornet continued to burrow deeper into my wrist, eventually making its way into my forearm, my belly started to burn. Even though the nurse said it looked fine, the line was no longer pumping narcotics into my vein every six minutes, it was pumping them into my skin and surrounding tissue. I wasn't getting any pain relief but I was developing my first complication.

When the unnamed nurse finally returned with my ice pack, she found my husband and I distraught. Compassion was slowly culled from so many of my colleagues, and the pandemic brought the worst out of all of us. I am appalled and ashamed to have experienced firsthand how deadly it is when support staff, and residents can't accommodate their patient load. While I am frustrated by the unnamed nurses and floating staff who dismissed me, I don't exactly blame them.

So, who's to blame?

Big Medicine, the conglomeration of all our corporate overlords, is the concept of profits over patients, numbers over natural remedies, and growth margins over genuine connections. Gone are the days of the good old country doctor for they have been replaced by nameless interns, residents that rotate, and a cast of clinicians who are more burnout than any previous generation.

This first nurse was an example of that burnout. She was so nonchalant about my pain because she was overworked and stuck on a floor that was understaffed. She didn't have time to care. I knew this type of work ethic was likely having experienced burnout myself and so I prepared for that by bringing snacks for the staff. We brought bags of Dove chocolate and when I was unconscious, my husband put them in a nice bowl at the door so anyone coming or going could grab a sweet treat.

Not even chocolate could help me.

When she returned with the ice, she dismissed me again, "It's fine."

"No, it's…an infiltrate." I argued back finding my words.

I didn't have a chance to argue with her further because it was a shift change. Thankfully, the next nurse that came in to relieve her agreed with my initial assessment: it was an infiltrate. I didn't have the energy or the words to advocate for myself by the time she came on shift and I felt myself slipping in and out of consciousness just to escape the pain. The IV was eventually replaced seven times over the course of those first ten days hospitalized. My veins kept failing and I was running out of places to run fluids and medications.

Despite the surgery, I was still struggling to eat and the nausea was unbearable. When the nurses did arrive with my oral medications, they would be up to two hours late. When I complained about the pain management, I was flagged as a drug seeker. As the hours turned into days, instant after instant of negligence piled up culminating in me falling in the bathroom, unattended, and left alone for several hours.

My husband was furious. He was at his breaking point so when a nurse admitted to us that she turned off my call button so I would stop paging her, he demanded an alternative nurse to replace her. He stood up at my bedside, quiet anger in his voice, as he squeezed my shoulder protectively. I put my hand to my husband's chest, looking up at him and begging him to sit down. I knew if he showed too much emotion, hospital staff would remove him from my room and bar him from returning.

I warned him, "Stop, they'll never listen if you get angry."

I wasn't wrong.

Shortly after this exchange, a representative from the hospital came into my room to address my husband. She identified herself as a Patient Advocate. She was a thin woman with coiffed blonde hair and she had a nasty habit of sitting on my bed next to me. I was in so much pain, I didn't want anyone touching me, never mind a stranger who was there to enforce hospital policy, and each rustle of my bed she made caused worsening spikes of nausea.

I asked if she was there to help advocate for me or for the hospital.

I told her that the pain management was delayed by hours, the multiple IV infiltrates, and that no one had helped me shower or so much as sponge bath, and that I was left unattended and fell in the bathroom. She nodded and admitted those concerns were "serious," but she was there to advocate for the hospital staff after my husband threatened their safety.

According to her, I was considered an aggressive and noncompliant patient and my husband was deemed a risk to hospital staff. She stated she was there to defuse him as a security threat and to escort him off the premises if he didn't "behave."

"Are you joking?" I asked, flabbergasted.

She responded, "My staff doesn't find it funny when he threatens them."

"My husband didn't threaten anyone," I countered.

Before we could say anything more, the patient advocate stated, "It's only by my good graces he's allowed in this building right now".

295

The patient advocate said she would give us some time to discuss our options. After talking it over as a family, we agreed that my mother should come and take his place as my daily visitor today. The advocate said he was allowed to come every other day, but only during daylight hours, and only if he behaved. We agreed because we had no other options. My mother understood how to talk to doctors more than he did. This wasn't her first rodeo when it came to medical staff treating her like an inconvenience, and she was able to speak up when I couldn't.

And I really couldn't speak up effectively.

All I could do was curl up and keep hitting that damn drug button.

It only takes about seventy-two hours for the human body to become dependent on opioids. I was on that Dilaudid pump for nearly ten days in that first hospital. I found myself quickly addicted but in the microcosm that is an inpatient hospital room, drug use just hits differently. On one hand, the oral medications were never on time but on the other, once my IV was restored I was able to hit that button and get short acting, quick relief.

It seemed that the general surgery recovery floor had no fucks left to give for unconventional surgeries like mine, and they looked at me as someone who was having a histrionic reaction to a standard procedure. When in reality, my surgery was complicated and required close management. To summarize, my medical team did the following:

1. Sedated the patient (me!)
2. Opened an incision in the abdomen from the ribs to the belly button.

3. Used metal retractors to hold the various organs out of the way to expose the anterior aspect of the spinal column.
4. Isolated the Median Arcuate Ligament and the necrotic nerve bundle entrapping the artery and vein.
5. Cut the Median Arcuate Ligament, freeing the vasculature!
6. Dissect out the necrotic and damaged nerve fibers from the Celiac ganglion.
7. Close 'er back up!
8. Pray.

There was a lot of moving around in there, so it's no wonder my body was a mess of gas, chemicals, and emotions. Each day I got a little stronger, but my body still didn't feel right. I felt like a rubber band had bisected me and, every time I tried to uncurl my spine, it wanted to snap right back in place. The oozing incision eventually split midway through, resulting in a gape that I couldn't look directly at for fear of fainting.

I didn't want to look inside myself.

The incision was reinforced with surgical glue and steri-strips, no different than a superficial laceration I'd repair in my office on a spitting toddler, and I was counseled on the importance of eating, walking, and positive thinking! I ate meager bites of mashed potatoes and called that a success. Each day, I slid deeper and deeper into a narcotic haze. I'd hit that button every six minutes and pray for another gift from Hypnos. I didn't want to be awake. Everything felt like fire and hornets and, even though I was supposed to eat, I couldn't stop the waves of nausea that were worse than before I went under the knife.

Was this all a mistake? What have I done to myself?

My best distraction was, once again, medical television. As I was hooked up to my drip, I decided to mainline every episode of "Doped," the true story of the rise and fall of Purdue Pharma and the oxycodone crisis they created in the United States. Sometime around my seventh day in the hospital, I took a hit from my pump and my heart started to feel funny. It felt like it did when I was in the psych ward; it was beating way too fast but something else felt off about it. It made me feel floppy. My husband was at my bedside and told the residents something was wrong with me when they rotated through that afternoon.

I wasn't getting enough food in me and I still hadn't had a bowel movement so I suspected an electrolyte deficiency causing heart complications. I told them as much, requesting bloodwork to check my sugar, potassium, and magnesium. The residents discussed my request amongst themselves, but said no bloodwork was needed until the next morning. They said the surgeon didn't like extra labs drawn on patients, so I'd have to wait.

Except, I didn't make it to the morning.

Minutes before visiting hours ended, the pain in my chest worsened acutely. I clutched my heart, head flopping forward as weakness consumed me. The yellow sensation of sickness started to thicken around the corners of my eyes but when I tried to talk, I couldn't get the words out.

My husband jumped to attention and called for help in the hallway. This time, he wasn't flagged as aggressive because something was very wrong and the nursing staff knew it. Someone called for a crash cart.

The residents were paged and outside I heard one of them say, "Is she seizing?"

I felt my eyes swimming from yellow into blackness, but the next thing I remember is the resident calling off the code with relieved laughter, and patting me heartily on my back. He told me I scared them but nothing was wrong, it was just a "dramatic presentation."

Dramatic presentation of what though? I screamed internally, too weak to argue.

My husband asked if he just witnessed a seizure.

They told him not to worry about it.

He went home that night without any resolution because he wasn't allowed to stay past dark. It is rare that the trauma of our witnesses gets acknowledged. He watched as my world expanded and shrunk before our very eyes but was overwhelmingly powerless. We both were. The next day, we asked for a transfer to a closer hospital after my morning blood work showed dangerously low levels of potassium and magnesium. If either of those electrolytes get too low you're looking at complications like abnormal heart rhythms (hello QT syndrome!), seizures, and death. I knew in my repaired gut the longer I stayed at this hospital, the more likely I would be to keep having hospital induced complications.

We were informed that, if I were to transfer, my medical team would have no further contact with me and my case would be dismissed by the vascular surgeon.

Cue the feelings of abandonment.

Bounce Back

The day I was discharged from the hospital, I felt like I was breaking out of a prison.

I had not hit my goals for discharge but my surgeon did not protest when I asked to be sent home. The patient advocate even stopped by to wish me well on the way out, which I found particularly patronizing. I wasn't leaving the hospital happy, even though she said that was her goal, I was breaking out because I didn't trust them to keep me safe during a difficult postoperative period. Even though I had not been eating solid food, was not tolerating oral pain medication, and I had not been able to bathe myself once since the surgery (ten days prior!), they let me leave.

The nursing staff unhooked me from the Dilaudid drip, handed me a packet of papers, and told me not to miss my one week follow up with my vascular surgeon at his outpatient office. I could barely keep my head up but, as the attendant wheeled me down to the first floor of the hospital, I was desperate to rip off my mask and take that first deep breath of fresh, spring air.

The blast of cold was invigorating, but my body felt so very far away, it barely registered when they propped me up into the passenger side of the seat and closed the door leaving me to my husband in the driver's seat.

"You OK?" My husband looked worried.

He wasn't convinced I should be going home, but I smiled weakly and asked if we could keep the windows down for the car ride home. I told him I wanted to see my puppy and sleep in my bed. I promised as soon as we got home, I'd take some medicine and drink some water.

I cried as he drove over bumps in the road, quietly holding my freshly sliced belly. I was due for my first dose of pain medication within four hours of discharge, but even with the addition of my vaporized cannabis on the comfort of my couch, I couldn't hold liquids down never mind pills. I could barely hold my head up because my electrolytes were crashing and I was experiencing the beginning stages of opioid withdrawal.

My body grew hot, then cold, then wet as it shook with chills.

My stomach started to heave, but nothing was inside, and the outside threatened to burst open.

My muscles started to ache, visibly twitching under pale skin, and I begged for unconsciousness.

The hours passed and I was unable to move from my position on the couch. I couldn't so much as sip water. My beloved dog Pippin watched worried from his space on the floor. He was desperate to hop up on the couch next to me and nuzzle me, and he didn't understand why he needed to stay away. We couldn't risk his fur getting into the incision, or his exuberance knocking me down. I could barely lift my head to acknowledge him. So, when the ambulance was finally called in the early morning hours the next day and the cherry berry lights were flashing outside, my dog cried in his kennel, mirroring my whimpers. My father and mother stood outside our apartment door frame in pajamas, too afraid to move, but looking onward fearful they were watching their daughter die.

I remember my husband begging the EMTs to be careful as they carried me down the steps and watching his face disappear as they closed the vehicle doors with a loud slam.

My heart rate wouldn't go below 150 beats per minute and my EKG was showing signs of QT prolongation. The QT interval measures the time it takes for the lower heart chambers, the ventricles, to contract and relax. While grossly oversimplified, our electrolytes control our heart's ability to safely beat and if they remain unstable, this arrhythmia can develop. Patients can be asymptomatic or they can endorse dizziness, fluttering of the heart (we call those palpitations in medicine), and in severe cases seizures and death.

As the eighth IV of the week entered the crook of my right arm, I cried to the ER physician for relief, and he whispered his condolences as he validated my complications. After eleven days of not being listened to by my surgical team, this man was an angel at my bedside. He reassured me he would work on a transfer back to my surgical hospital.

Except that didn't happen.

It took fourteen hours for the small town hospital to figure out what to do with me because my vascular surgeon refused to accept me as a bounce back. In medicine, a bounce back is when a patient is discharged from the hospital but "bounces back" with complications in under 48 hours. Officially, the vascular surgery team stated I was experiencing an unrelated medical condition that was not within their scope and I was discharged from their care when I decided to leave the day prior.

Eventually, an ambulance transferred me back to the place I was born thirty-five years earlier and the place I lost my mind the year prior. Once established as a patient on the twenty-second floor of this hospital, the receiving care team wanted to rule out a blood clot in my chest. I was sent for an emergency angiogram and ultrasound of my chest and abdomen.

In order for the ultrasound tech to check my incision, she needed to apply cold gel and the transducer directly onto the scar and push down and around. I didn't want her to touch me. I knew I needed these tests but I couldn't stop hyperventilating. I managed to squeak out a few words explaining I was having a panic attack, to which she calmly took my hand and patted me.

"I won't do anything until you're ready," She reassured me.

I admitted I thought my constant retching surely undid all the surgeon's work. I was afraid of what we would learn once we did the imaging studies. She didn't rush me past my emotions to get the test done, she listened. This is called holding space for someone and she held space for me by leading me through a series of breathing exercises. She validated my fear and verbalized that it was terrifying to have an ultrasound and to have someone pushing down on your belly when you just had surgery, *and* that it had to be done but she would be as gentle as possible.

She squeezed my hand while I squeezed hers. I let the tears go and I consented to the tests.

Thankfully, the ultrasound showed no damage was sustained and the angiogram which followed immediately after was negative for a clot. They took me back up to my room, which was a private room, and advised me the next morning the rounding gastroenterologist would meet me and discuss my case. I slept fitfully because my heart was still jack-hammering throughout the early morning hours.

When morning finally came, the gastroenterologist that walked into my room wasn't a stranger. After nearly twenty years, Fate decided to bring me my original treating doctor from childhood. The doctor that stood in front of my bed rounding with a gaggle of medical students was once the man that prescribed my Imuran, that conducted my pediatric liver biopsies, and that treated me for autoimmune hepatitis for nearly a decade.

He started to introduce himself, not once looking up from his clipboard, but I interrupted him with a dry laugh, "Remember me?"

He didn't. In an attempt to identify myself I pulled my rat's nests of a braid out from behind my smock because he would always compliment my hair way back when.

"I don't have Autoimmune Hepatitis this time," I shrugged.

He didn't bite because he didn't remember me. He wasn't even curious in the slightest! I will never understand doctors who lose that spark and, when I got his bill a few months later for nearly $500 dollars for five minutes of his time, I was angry. He didn't properly diagnose me decades ago, he barely acknowledged me as an inpatient, and yet here he was collecting another round of copays for little more than a signature.

He confirmed that my magnesium, potassium, and sodium were dangerously low and that I needed IV supplementation of those minerals to restore my heart function. He also shared that my imaging showed no damage to the underlying surgery, no evidence of hernias or internal bleeding, and no blood clots. But because the QT prolongation put me at risk of developing a deadly heart rhythm, we needed to immediately discontinue any medications that could contribute to the abnormality. This included all narcotics.

I was advised that because my case was so complicated, the Head of Gastroenterology would be by later to discuss my options for transitioning off the cocktail of drugs that put me at risk. The Head of Gastroenterology was a well-esteemed physician in his nineties and he had been practicing for longer than I had been alive.

When this physician entered the room, his white hair gleaming like a halo under the fluorescent lights, he was flanked by two medical students. I was immediately impressed when he sat down next to me, and the students sat in the chairs in front of me, so we could all talk at my eye level.

He treated me as his equal even though he didn't know anything about me personally. It wasn't until after he left I was struck with the realization we could have been colleagues. Just before I accepted my urgent care position, I had an interview to work with his practice. I turned down that job because it was less lucrative than urgent care, but once I was on the receiving end of his bedside manner, I knew it would have been a fulfilling job.

I thought my surgeon was my savior, but this man with his kind eyes and kinder bedside manner was the physician priest I had been praying for all along. Together, we came up with a plan to get me out of the hospital and home. He answered my secular prayers and offered me both salve and salvation and together, we decided to stop all my medications except for IV Valium and rectal Tylenol because it was the only way to save my heart.

"Nausea is the worst thing you can experience. It serves no purpose," he admitted sagely, patting my hand just like the ultrasound tech before he left me to the nursing staff.

I've never been as scared as I was lying in the bed, wondering if the bags of IV magnesium and potassium would save me. Despite supplementation, my potassium and magnesium continued to plummet, and we considered the placement of a PICC line that would feed intravenous nutrition directly into my chest. I didn't want that. I didn't want anything. I just wanted the pain to stop. I don't entirely remember what happened next, but I *do* remember praying to Death, as the yellow haze of illness threatened to swallow my entire existence.

Prayer for the Surviving Dying

This chapter is a selection of journal excerpts and poems written while laying in the hospital bed as my body continued to shut down after surgery.

In these ramblings, I beg for Death to release me from my hospital bed and then I beg Death for just one more chance. After my physician priest offered me a plan, the tone of the journal changes into one of desperate hope.

Inspired by opioid withdrawal and electrolyte imbalances, this is my most intimate secular prayer.

It's also an invitation to you.

It is an invitation to you to keep going, because you never know what's going to happen next. Sometimes, your secular prayers are answered.

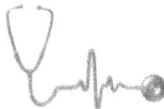

And so we gather here today to say a prayer for the surviving dying.

We gather today.

I've lost count of how many things have been put inside me as someone who has become rather proficient at surviving dying.

I can't keep track of the tubes and the moves that have been made inside my own body, but I do know I want it to be over.

There's a strange sensation that comes from dancing with death once too many times;

there's a familiarity that stalks you from inside your own ventricles.

It's comforting, almost, to let the waning beat of your heart drum guide you to a place where there's no need to sway again.

To be silent.

To sleep.

To succeed in giving up the ghost has a pull that can't be ignored.

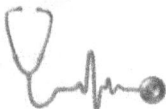

Dancing with death is something people romanticize, but for me, it was more of a silent partner I knew I had to fall back on.

Once you say die, it's always an option.

Illness that blooms in childhood has deep roots and, as each layer of adulthood approaches and passes me over, I can't help but wonder if this life is a shallow example of what it means to truly be alive.

Instead of planning futures and building a world of my own, I'm left recounting the setbacks and watching from the sidelines.

As my family and friends move on, I remain ghosted in this life, fighting for just a small stronghold, a foothold really, in which I can pause and catch my broken breath.

I stopped dreaming of hope a long time ago and, the longer my body decays while my heart still beats,

The darker my prayers become.

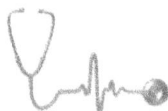

Sometimes, when the pain of being inside this mauled body gets to be too much, I'll say a prayer to my beloved Death.

I'd beg him to release me from these traps of sensation and sorrow.

Most often these prayers take place in the bathroom, a place of respite, where tears and shit and fear mix together in the most private of places.

There is sanctity in shit.

There is divinity in crying against a cold tile floor.

There is nothing that can replace the altar of indoor pipes and water that can wash away your sins if only you make it to the basin in time.

I'd light candles in my mind,

Create burning bonfires of single stalks, smoke rising up in earnest, following the smoke until it lifted me up and away from this place and into the great beyond.

Take me away.

Take me away now.

Please.

And so I pray.

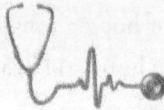

My mother once said to me that I didn't believe in prayer.

It wasn't an unkind or judgmental statement, but rather an observation from her limited perspective.

Her prayers went to different gods, though many overlap.

She shared this at my bedside as I struggled to keep my hammering heart in check.

With each toss and turn in the bed, my heartbeat thrummed within my ears, pounding an ancient rhythm that said:

"Your prayers will be answered soon."

But I'm not ready yet.

Please, I'm not ready yet.

I thought I was.

I thought I wanted to be released into smoke and ash and ascension, but I'm not ready yet.

I want to go home:

I want to build bonfires of candles set to other stories and other secular prayers.

I want to learn how to dance with the other deities that have always been waiting in the wings.

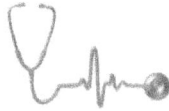

To my Dear Death:

I do not discard you.

I honor you for what you offer, but I beg for a different release:

Release me to dance with the others.

Release me to take hands with hope.

Release me to feel the relief of tranquility and the soothing steps of serenity.

Take me away.

Take me away now.

And so I pray.

We throw ourselves onto the altar of alternative hope

Basking in the gory glory of the stories of the deities who died before us

Begging as we break bread to remain above ground

Secretly searching for the sacred that never was and never will be

Because as long as we throw ourselves to the ground

Because as long as we throw ourselves down

One more time

One more time

We might have one more time.

Life After Diagnosis

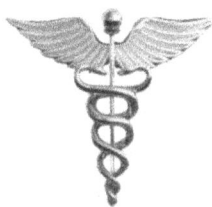

Do You Need More Dilaudid?

"Do you need more Dilaudid?"

It was my first time seeing the vascular surgeon since I was discharged from his hospital. We hadn't even spoken since he refused to take my case as a bounce back with medical complications.

At this point, I had been discharged from the second hospital after successfully surviving acute opioid withdrawal and QT prolongation from polypharmacy. I was tolerating small bites of food and water and the Head of Gastroenterology signed off on me using inhaled THC and Tylenol for pain management outpatient. There was no judgment from the physician priest, only sage understanding and I promised myself I would channel his wisdom once I got back into my own medical practice.

Sitting in the small office with the vascular surgeon who saved my life, I felt conflicted by my experience with him. On one hand, objectively the resection of the Median Arcuate Ligament improved my symptoms and I was eating again for the first time in years. He validated a lifetime of pain as a physical deformity and didn't gaslit me into thinking my pain was all in my head, but he also didn't really care about anything other than the actual pathology.

He asked me again as he pushed on the thick keloidal scar, "Do you need anything for pain?"

He scowled, feeling the fibrous band of tissue. He wasn't happy with the amount of scar tissue but I loved my scar. My scar was proof I survived a battle and even though I was gaslit by other providers for years, all I had to do now was lift my shirt and show off a four-inch scar. I was proud of my proof.

"No, it triggered QT prolongation." I responded just as flatly, staring at him from under my fogged-up glasses. "I'm just using Tylenol and THC."

He did a double take, "That's it? No Dilaudid? No ketorolac? Nothing else?"

"No, I had too many complications with it…" I started but he cut me off, ready to move onto the next patient.

He closed his computer, "I'm sorry you had a difficult post op period, but as I warned you, every case is different." He paused before continuing, "I'm glad you're doing better now. Just make sure you follow up with your primary care provider."

As he was walking out the door, I asked, "What about physical therapy? And our post op photo?"

"I'll have my receptionist give you a script." He walked out the door but I followed him, asking if I could have a picture of the two of us in front of his map of patients.

After a successful surgery, MALS patients were invited to put a push pin into their geographical location on his wall of maps. Hundreds of push pins were scattered across the globe and as he put his arm around me, I realized I was part of a community of reconstructed bodies that he touched. I was part of something so much larger than myself. Every single one of those push pins had their own story filled with triumphs and tragedies.

I took my pin, number 651, and I placed it in the city where I was born.

We took our picture and we shook hands, saying our final goodbyes. I asked him if he ever considered publishing his experiences in medical journals or speaking at conferences so other clinicians could learn from his expertise. He shook his head and said he had enough on his plate. He had no desire to publish at this time. But someone needed to publish these stories. Someone needed to start speaking for this community from both sides of the exam table.

On my way out, I asked for copies of my medical chart to keep for my own records because I knew I wouldn't be returning to his office again any time soon. He didn't offer post operative care beyond what was just done and my primary care provider didn't even believe in MALS in the first place, so I was left to my own devices in the postoperative period.

I also took that prescription for physical therapy. Later, when I read through my medical chart I was amazed to realize nowhere in those documents did it truly describe the experiences I had while inpatient. Sure, it detailed the procedure, all the nursing notes were in there and the values of low electrolytes but a medical record is not the same thing as your medical story, and it will never fully encapsulate your life, death, and diagnoses in between.

As I read my medical records I realized not only did I survive, but I was also uniquely posed to start communicating between the worlds of patient and provider as a survivor of vascular compression surgery. There was a lot of work to do for my fellow Zebras and I was ready.

It was time to start writing.

When A Clinician (Finally) Calls Out

"I can't come to work today." I texted my regional manager.

It was exactly 173 days after my MALS reconstruction surgery, and I was back at my Urgent Care practicing medicine four days a week. The surgery was successful, but I wasn't normal, nor would I ever be entirely normal ever again. I was still subject to flares and needed to be gentle with my body during them. I held my breath, waiting for her inevitable response. Another wave of nausea gripped me and I vomited mucus onto the towel lining my bathroom floor.

"Is there any chance you can come in later today? If you don't, we'll have to close both clinics." My regional manager responded via text.

Her response was filled with subtext: If you don't show up, no one will get paid and patients will suffer. This is not an uncommon dilemma for medical providers and it's even more pronounced in the retail urgent care industry: if we get sick, who looks after our patients? I looked up at the sky, praying for an answer, and asked myself what I would tell a patient in a similar situation: how would I counsel them?

I would counsel them to take a sick day, curl up in the bedroom with a hot pad, take their prescribed medication, and hydrate. I would counsel them to enforce boundaries with their employer because:

Sick people can't heal sick people.

My employer doesn't need to know the specifics of my health conditions, but in America, we often sacrifice our medical privacy for a modicum of understanding. The sad thing is, the chronically ill are rarely understood, and, unless we are productive (like a clinician that can take in high numbers on an outpatient shift), then we are dismissed as "bad employees."

The implicit meaning in the text from my boss suggested I take additional ownership in the clinic for support staff: it is my responsibility to keep it staffed no matter what.

Except, it's not.

I responded to my regional manager, "I wouldn't call out if I didn't need to; I'm sorry but I can't come in today."

I considered the matter closed, took my medication, and fell asleep for a few hours. When I woke up, I was surprised to see several missed phone calls and a variety of text messages asking for clarification on various patients.

The next day I wasn't feeling any better.

I texted my regional once more, déjà vu washing over me, "I can't believe I'm doing this again and I'm so sorry, but I need to call out sick today too."

This time the response was more intimidating: "I hope you feel better but this time we need a doctor's note."

I responded quickly, referencing state law which outlines that employers can only ask for a note explaining three consecutive days off of work in a row. I had not called out multiple days in a row, but I did realize it was a holiday weekend, Labor Day to be exact. I understood she was suspicious, but I wasn't trying to score a day down by the lake; I was just trying to get my symptoms under control so I could get off the toilet.

My regional responded, "It's a holiday weekend."

Staring back at the black mirror, I refused to back down. "Based on what policy do you need that documentation?"

My heart pounded waiting for a response, but the funny thing is, she never responded. I called her bluff. And I didn't drag my tired self to go sit in a waiting room where someone less qualified than I would nod, agree with me that I was ill and needed the day off, and write me a performative note wasting their time and mine. What I did was get back under those covers once my prescriptions kicked back in.

Over my medical career, I've seen support staff, medical assistants and receptionists, blue collar workers that lack the clout to call out, nurse their own illnesses in shame while on shift because the pressure to keep working is so high. When people scorn us, saying, "No one wants to work anymore," I can't help but laugh, and then cry, because I realize no one wants to work in these conditions anymore. We deserve better. We deserve to be treated like adults, not children trying to play hooky.

When I call out sick as a clinician, I am doing so because I know my body and I know the risks that I can and can't safely take. I will never put my patients at risk and, now that I know my worth, I won't continue to put myself at risk.

Consider this my white coat-endorsed professional opinion: If you think you need to take a day off to recover from an illness or injury, take the day off.

Let the corporate overlords figure out how to staff your absence.

That's their job, after all, not yours, even on holidays.

Love, Lady House

She barely had a fever, but my medical assistant shared that the patient was on three different antibiotics already, and was post-operative from a complicated double knee replacement. As she hobbled past my open office door, I did a quick visual exam and realized she was fairly unsteady on her feet, using two arm-brace crutches, but was cheerfully bantering with support staff.

Her chief complaint popped up on my urgent care screen: "COVID Rapid."

Her past medical history showed arthritis, but she was relatively young, having only passed her fiftieth birthday a few months earlier. She requested a panel of viral tests, Influenza A/B and COVID19, and I was happy to oblige as I quickly realized she was an autoimmune case. The big viruses du jour were ruled out, so we could proceed with our visit.

I introduced myself, conducted a focused physical examination, and proclaimed her early in the course of an acute viral common cold, but with precautions considering her post-op status.

"I don't understand how she could still get sick even if she's on three antibiotics," her husband lamented to no one in particular.

"That's actually a really great question." I gestured to my patient, "As you know, with autoimmune issues, we tend to present a bit out of the ordinary, so with a common cold, which is a virus not bacteria, you will take longer to recover from it, especially post op."

"I don't really know." She shrugged.

Confused, I asked, "But you have arthritis; I assume rheumatoid based on your age?"

"Yes, but I haven't really gotten any information yet," she said.

As I was originally diagnosed with rheumatoid arthritis and then autoimmune hepatitis and then gastroparesis and then complex post-traumatic stress disorder and then finally Median Arcuate Ligament Syndrome, my heart ached for her. I knew the road she was traveling and to be early in the diagnosis process can be scary if you don't have someone holding your hand. I told her a little bit about my story, this story, and how to advocate for herself at her follow up specialist appointments. I also demonstrated my first symptom of autoimmunity, opening and closing my right hand slowly, mimicking the crunching, clicking range of motion I experienced as a fifteen-year-old patient.

Her eyes opened wide, and she slapped her left thigh, just above the bandages and looked at her husband, "Do you remember when I was nineteen!?"

Her husband nodded emphatically, "You used to do that with your hands all the time!"

"Is it possible that I've had this my whole life? When I was nineteen I would wake up and my hands wouldn't close. I told my parents and my doctors, but no one listened."

Even though we were in the middle of an urgent care office, surrounded by cell phone providers, a fast-food chicken restaurant, and across from a megamart, for a moment we were two Zebras connecting, and I taught her what it meant to live with an autoimmune condition. Unexpectedly, I became the physician (assistant) priest she didn't know she needed and I realized I had a duty to care for others the way my physician priest cared for me. I taught her how to stand up for herself when other clinicians dismissed her, because they will, and I gave her my card in case she ever needed an urgent prayer answered.

"Thirty years. I've lived with this pain for thirty years." She shook her head in disbelief. "I'm so glad I met you. You've answered more about me than any doctor has ever been able to in a ten-minute visit for a COVID test."

We both laughed, and then we both cried just a little. If she had been properly diagnosed and placed on immunosuppressive therapy in time, she might not be battling twin infections in false joints before retirement. I know I can't save everyone, but I can share my tips and tricks for surviving dying one day at a time.

Later that night, when my husband asked how the clinic day went, I told him I had a great day and even had one of my "Lady House Moments", a phrase I use to describe moments where I connected with patients over an important medical detail others missed.

"You're not Lady House," My husband said, the two of us standing in the kitchen preparing a small meal of cantaloupe, cheese, and crackers, my resurrected body growling in hunger.

Before I could protest he continued, "House is what? House is a fictional character. He's a fantasy. You, you are real. You care about your patients, you pick up on things no one else thinks to look for, and you are a real fucking person. You are a giantess."

"I do? I am?" I asked quietly.

"You do. And you are. You actually saved yourself." He winked at me and popped another piece of cantaloupe in his mouth, offering me the other bite. "I was there, remember?"

Sometimes we need a witness to remind us that we survived the unsurvivable. My family acted as a witness for me and now I am acting as a witness for my patients by writing out their secular prayers of medicine one case at a time. As I continue to hold out a lantern for the other lost souls on the path to health and wellness, I offer these secular prayers as a reminder that hope is still alive as long as you are.

Once upon a time, I wanted to be saved from the horrors of a body that never fit, because I felt like a monster marred with pain.

But we were never monsters.

We are hypotheticals and, when hypotheticals happen, we always deserve dignity.

Notes on Sources

Rotting Out His Head:

Atlas SJ, Grant RW, Ferris TG, et al. *Patient-physician connectedness and quality of primary care. Annals of Internal Medicine* 2009; 150:325.

Ball, Jane RN, Joyce Dains FNP-BC, John A. Flynn MD, Barry S. Solomon MD, and Rosalyn W. Stewart MD. 2014. *Seidel's Guide to Physical Examination: An Interprofessional Approach (Mosby's Guide to Physical Examination)*. 8th ed. Mosby.

Zipkin DA, Umscheid CA, Keating NL, et al. *Evidence-based risk communication: a systematic review*. Annals of Internal Medicine 2014; 161:270.

Viagra Two Ways:

Loe, Meika. 2006. *The Rise of Viagra: How the Little Blue Pill Changed Sex in America*. 1st ed. NYU Press.

Nehra A, Jackson G, Miner M, et al. *The Princeton III Consensus recommendations for the management of erectile dysfunction and cardiovascular disease*. Mayo Clinic Proceeding 2012; 87:766.

Rampin O, Giuliano F. *Central control of the cardiovascular and erection systems: possible mechanisms and interactions.* American Journal of Cardiology 2000; 86:19F.

Circumcision Syncope

Caldwell, Brian T. MD. "Olympic Circumstraint." McArthurMedical.Com. McArthur Medical, November 3, 2020. https://mcarthurmedical.com/wp-content/uploads/2022/01/Olympic_Circumstraint_Datasheet_MMSI.pdf.

Horowitz M, Gershbein AB. *Gomco circumcision: When is it safe?* Journal of Pediatric Surgery 2001; 36:1047.

Omole F, Smith W, Carter-Wicker K. *Newborn Circumcision Techniques.* American Family Physician 2020; 101:680.

Overview of surgical devices. *In: Manual for Early Infant Male Circumcision Under Local Anesthesia*, World Health Organization (Ed), WHO Press, Geneva 2010. P.50.

Bechet Dump:

Cree BA, Khan O, Bourdette D, et al. *Clinical characteristics of African Americans vs Caucasian Americans with multiple sclerosis.* Neurology 2004; 63:2039.

Brownlee WJ, Hardy TA, Fazekas F, Miller DH. *Diagnosis of multiple sclerosis: progress and challenges.* Lancet 2017; 389:1336.

Eriksson M, Andersen O, Runmarker B. *Long-term follow up of patients with clinically isolated syndromes, relapsing-remitting and secondary progressive multiple sclerosis.* Multiple Sclerosis 2003; 9:260.

Mahr A, Belarbi L, Wechsler B, et al. *Population-based preva-lence study of Behçet's disease: dif erences by ethnic origin and low variation by age at immigration.* Arthritis & Rheumatol-ogy 2008; 58:3951.

Rice CM, Cottrell D, Wilkins A, Scolding NJ. *Primary pro-gressive multiple sclerosis: progress and challenges.* Journal of Neurology, Neurosurgery, and Psychiatry 2013; 84:1100.

Sakane T, Takeno M, Suzuki N, Inaba G. *Behçet's disease.* New England Journal of Medicine. 1999; 341:1284.

You Killed My Child:

Lee DM, Weinblatt ME. *Rheumatoid arthritis.* Lancet 2001; 358:903.

Lineker S, Badley E, Charles C, et al. *Defining morning stif ness in rheumatoid arthritis.* Journal of Rheumatology. 1999; 26:1052.

You Look Like Me:

National Commission on Correctional Health Care. *Stand-ards for Health Services in Correctional Facilities*, Chicago 2015.

National Commission on Correctional Health Care. *Stand-ards for Health Services in Prisons,* Chicago 2018.

Ndeffo-Mbah ML, Vigliotti VS, Skrip LA, et al. *Dynamic Models of Infectious Disease Transmission in Prisons and the General Population.* Epidemiology Review 2018; 40:40.

Prescribing Dream Control:

Camcevi (leuprolide mesylate) [prescribing information]. *Durham, NC: Accord BioPharma Inc; November 2022.*

Guay DR. *Drug treatment of paraphilic and nonparaphilic sexual disorders.* Clinical Therapeutics. 2009;31(1):1-31. doi:10.1016/j.clinthera.2009.01.009

D.I.D. I Do That?

Chu JA, Frey LM, Ganzel BL, Matthews JA. *Memories of childhood abuse: dissociation, amnesia, and corroboration.* American Journal of Psychiatry 1999; 156:749.

Ellason JW, Ross CA, Fuchs DL. *Lifetime axis I and II comorbidity and childhood trauma history in dissociative identity disorder.* Psychiatry 1996; 59:255.

Loewenstein RJ, Putnam FW. *The clinical phenomenology of males with multiple personality disorder.* Journal of Trauma & Dissociation 1990; 3:135.

Ross CA. *Epidemiology of multiple personality disorder and dissociation.* Psychiatric Clinics of North America. 1991; 14:503.

Spiegel D, Loewenstein RJ, Lewis-Fernández R, et al. *Dissociative disorders in DSM-5.* Depress Anxiety 2011; 28:824.

Autism Speaks For Itself:

"About Autism Speaks: Our Co-Founders." Autism Speaks. Autism Speaks, Accessed September 1, 2022.
https://www.autismspeaks.org/our-founders.

American Psychiatric Association. *Stereotypic movement disorder. In: Diagnostic and Statistical Manual of Mental Disorders,* Fifth, American Psychiatric Association, Arlington, VA 2013.

Cooper, John, Timothy Heron, and William Heward. 2019. *Applied Behavior Analysis.* 3rd ed. Pearson.

Falkmer T, Anderson K, Falkmer M, Horlin C. *Diagnostic procedures in autism spectrum disorders: a systematic literature review.* European Child and Adolescent Psychiatry 2013; 22:329.

Grandin, Temple, and Richard Panek. 2014. *The Autistic Brain: Helping Different Kinds of Minds Succeed.* Reprint.

Grandin, Temple, and Oliver Sacks. 2006. *Thinking in Pictures, Expanded Edition: My Life with Autism.* Vintage.

Price, Devon PHD. 2022. *Unmasking Autism: Discovering the New Faces of Neurodiversity.* 1st ed. Harmony.

Rosenblatt, Alan MD, and Paul Carbone MD. 2019. *Autism Spectrum Disorder: What Every Parent Needs to Know.* 1st ed. American Academy of Pediatrics.

Sheffer, Edith. 2020. *Asperger's Children: The Origins of Autism in Nazi Vienna.* 1st ed. W. W. Norton & Company.

Zwaigenbaum L, Bryson S, Lord C, et al. *Clinical assessment and management of toddlers with suspected autism spectrum disorder: insights from studies of high-risk infants.* Pediatrics 2009; 123:1383.

Because You're Nice To Me:
American Psychiatric Association. Diagnostic and Statistical Manual of Mental Disorders, Fifth Edition, Text Revision (DSM-5-TR), Washington, DC 2022.

ASHER R. *Munchausen's syndrome.* Lancet 1951; 1:339.

Jimenez XF, Nkanginieme N, Dhand N, et al. *Clinical, demographic, psychological, and behavioral features of factitious disorder: A retrospective analysis.* General Hospital Psychiatry 2020; 62:93.

Krahn LE, Li H, O'Connor MK. *Patients who strive to be ill: factitious disorder with physical symptoms.* American Journal of Psychiatry 2003; 160:1163.

Is That Blood?

Weaver DH, Maxwell JG, Castleton KB. *Mallory-Weiss syndrome.* American Journal of Surgery 1969; 118:887.

Meeting Your Maker:

Damania, Zubin MD. *"Say Something (We Won't Give Up On You)."* ZDoggMD. September 16, 2017. Video: https://www.youtube.com/watch?v=-ZGpp0wESxw.

The Giantess, Me:

Adams JA, Farst KJ, Kellogg ND. *Interpretation of Medical Findings in Suspected Child Sexual Abuse: An Update for 2018.* Journal of Pediatric & Adolescent Gynecology 2018; 31:225.

Allen B. *Children with Sexual Behavior Problems: Clinical Characteristics and Relationship to Child Maltreatment.* Child Psychiatry & Human Development 2017; 48:189.

Filan, Misoo. "The Giantess." Misoo.Org. Accessed September 10, 2020.

https://www.misoo.org/the-giant-asian-gilrs.

Kaplow JB, Hall E, Koenen KC, et al. *Dissociation predicts later attention problems in sexually abused children.* Child Abuse & Neglect 2008; 32:261.

Trickett PK, Noll JG, Putnam FW. *The impact of sexual abuse on female development: lessons from a multigenerational, longitudinal research study.* Developmental Psychopathology 2011; 23:453.

Ice Cream Conspiracy:

Graham BS. *Rapid COVID-19 vaccine development.* Science 2020; 368:945.

Thompson MG, Stenehjem E, Grannis S, et al. Effectiveness of Covid-19 Vaccines in Ambulatory and Inpatient Care Settings. N Engl J Med 2021; 385:1355.

Travis J. Origins. *On the origin of the immune system.* Science 2009; 324:580.

Krammer F. *SARS-CoV-2 vaccines in development.* Nature 2020; 586:516.

Seven Days of Insanity:

Freudenreich O, Schulz SC, Goff DC. *Initial medical workup of first-episode psychosis: a conceptual review.* Early Interventional Psychiatry 2009; 3:10.

Manschreck TC. Delusional disorder. In: *The Spectrum of Psychotic Disorders: Neurobiology, Etiology, and Pathogeneses*, Fujii D, Ahmed I (Eds), Cambridge University Press, Cambridge 2007. P.116

Manschreck TC. The assessment of paranoid features. Comprehensive Psychiatry 1979; 20:370.

Sadock BJ, Sadock VA, Kaplan HI. *Kaplan and Sadock's Comprehensive Textbook of Psychiatry*, Lippincott Williams & Wilkins, 2009. Vol 1.

If the Shoe Fits:

Greys Anatomy: Everyday Angel. American Broadcasting Company, 2018.

Lipshutz B. A Composite Study of the Coelic Axis Artery. Annals of Surgery 1917; 65:159.

Kim EN, Lamb K, Relles D, et al. *Median Arcuate Ligament Syndrome-Review of This Rare Disease.* JAMA Surg 2016; 151:471.

Stiles-Shields C, Skelly CL, Mak GZ, et al. Psychological Factors and Outcomes in the Surgical Treatment of Pediatric Patients With Median Arcuate Ligament Syndrome. J Pediatr Gastroenterol Nutr 2018; 66:866.

Celiac Block Rock:

Sachdev AH, Gress FG. Celiac Plexus Block and Neurolysis: A Review. Gastrointest Gastrointestinal Endoscopy Clinics of North America 2018; 28:579.

The Resurrectionist:

Jimenez JC, Harlander-Locke M, Dutson EP. *Open and laparoscopic treatment of median arcuate ligament syndrome.* Journal of Vascular Surgery 2012; 56:869.

Roach, Mary. 2021. *Stif : The Curious Lives of Human Cadavers.* 1st ed. W. W. Norton & Company.

Bounce Back:

Moss AJ. *Long QT Syndrome.* JAMA 2003; 289:2041.

Roden DM. *Drug-induced prolongation of the QT interval.* New England Journal of Medicine 2004; 350:1013.

Yu H, Zhang L, Liu J, et al. *Acquired long QT syndrome in hospitalized patients.* Heart Rhythm 2017; 14:974.

Acknowledgements

You never know what words or what actions will impact another and this collection has been an astounding testimony to the pure magic and mayhem that is humanity.

Thank you to my family and my friends, to every reader, every clinician, every allied health professional, every patient, every creative, and every person who crossed their path with mine during the development of this book:

Please know I will be forever in your debt for saving my life.

You know who you are.

Writer, educator, public speaker, and Physician Assistant, Kateland Kelly knows what it is like to practice from both sides of the exam table. Practicing medicine since 2010, she combines a sense of humor that can only be honed through living life with chronic illness with a keen medical practice focused on putting her patients lived experiences first.

Her writing focuses on empowering patients and providers alike with clear communication because she believes the more we talk about conditions normally left in the dark, the lighter we will all become.